# Transforming Health Care

# Transforming Health Care

*Creating Equitable, Antiracist Healthcare Organizations*

LYNNE D. RICHARDSON, MD
AND
SIMA RABINOWITZ

*Foreword by*
CAMARA PHYLLIS JONES, MD, PHD, MPH

OXFORD
UNIVERSITY PRESS

OXFORD
UNIVERSITY PRESS

Oxford University Press is a department of the University of Oxford.
It furthers the University's objective of excellence in research, scholarship,
and education by publishing worldwide. Oxford is a registered trade mark of
Oxford University Press in the UK and in certain other countries.

Published in the United States of America by Oxford University Press
198 Madison Avenue, New York, NY 10016, United States of America.



Library of Congress Cataloging-in-Publication Data
Names: Richardson, Lynne D. author | Rabinowitz, Sima A. author
Title: Transforming health care : creating equitable, antiracist
healthcare organizations / Lynne D. Richardson, MD, and Sima Rabinowitz.
Description: New York, NY : Oxford University Press, [2026] |
Includes bibliographical references and index. |
Identifiers: LCCN 2025042965 (print) | LCCN 2025042966 (ebook) |
ISBN 9780197805374 paperback | ISBN 9780197805381 epub |
ISBN 9780197805404 ebook
Subjects: LCSH: Discrimination in medical care—United States |
Racism in medicine—United States | Social medicine—United States |
Minorities—Medical care—United States | Anti-racism—United States |
Health and race—United States
Classification: LCC RA563.M56 R53 2026 (print) | LCC RA563.M56 (ebook)
LC record available at https://lccn.loc.gov/2025042965
LC ebook record available at https://lccn.loc.gov/2025042966

DOI: 10.1093/oso/9780197805374.001.0001

Printed by Marquis Book Printing, Canada

The manufacturer's authorized representative in the EU for product safety is
Oxford University Press España S.A. of Parque Empresarial San Fernando de Henares,
Avenida de Castilla, 2 – 28830 Madrid (www.oup.es/en or product.safety@oup.com).
OUP España S.A. also acts as importer into Spain of products made by the manufacturer.

FSC
www.fsc.org
MIX
Paper | Supporting
responsible forestry
FSC® C103567

# Contents

# Foreword

## Transforming Health Care: Creating Equitable, Antiracist Healthcare Organizations

*Camara Phyllis Jones, MD, PhD, MPH*

Congratulations on opening this book! Your curiosity about the possibility of creating equitable, antiracist healthcare organizations in the United States will be bountifully satisfied by concrete examples and actionable strategies. I share the following definitions and frameworks to help ground your journey to support social justice and advance health equity.

### What is health equity?

Health equity is assurance of the conditions for optimal health for all people. Achieving health equity requires valuing all individuals and populations equally, recognizing and rectifying historical injustices, and providing resources according to need. Health disparities will be eliminated when health equity is achieved. Racism is a monumental barrier to achieving health equity in the United States.

### What is racism?

Racism is a system of structuring opportunity and assigning value based on the social interpretation of how one looks (which is what we call "race") that unfairly disadvantages some individuals and communities, unfairly advantages other individuals and communities, and saps the strength of the whole society through the waste of human resources.

Racism is foundational in the history of the United States. Racism continues to exist and have profoundly negative impacts on the health and well-being of our nation. Indeed, racism is the root cause of the myriad "race"-associated differences in health outcomes that we continue to document in this country across organ systems, age groups, and time. Why do I say this?

People are not born with a "race." People are born with parents who pass on their genes. They grow up in families in which they acquire language, access material resources, and learn patterns of behavior. They live in communities with specific histories, values, and creative cultures. Genetic ancestry, language, social class, culture—none of these things is "race."

However, these parents, families, and communities also exist in larger social contexts, which are too often characterized by systems of hierarchy. If people are born into a "race"-conscious society like the United States, one that notices differences in skin color, facial features, and hair texture; divides people into groups based on those physical characteristics; and calls those groups "race," then people are *assigned* a "race." This socially assigned "race" is not biology. This socially assigned "race" is not even permanent across geography or time. Indeed, for every reader of these words, there is some other place on this earth where your so-called "race" would be quite different from how you are living it today.

"Race" is a social construct used to subjugate individuality to a group identity in a "race"-based social hierarchy. "Race" is the substrate on which racism operates day to day in our "race"-conscious society to differentially structure opportunity and assign value. Racism, not some fictive biological "race," is the root cause of race-associated differences in health outcomes in the United States.

## How can racism impact health?

Racism impacts health on at least three levels: structural, personally mediated, and internalized. The interventions described in this book are primarily intended to address structural racism. Indeed, as illustrated in my often told *Gardener's Tale*, addressing personally mediated racism and/or internalized racism without addressing structural racism is likely to be ineffective in producing sustainable change.

Structural racism is "the system," the constellation of structures, policies, practices, norms, and values that, taken together, result in differential access to the goods, services, and opportunities of society by "race." Structural racism does not require an identifiable perpetrator because it has been institutionalized in our laws, customs, and background norms. Structural racism often shows up as inherited disadvantage and its reciprocal, inherited advantage. Manifestations include differences by "race" in material conditions and in access to power.

Examples of differences in material conditions include differential access by race to quality housing, excellent educational opportunities, equal employment opportunities, or even equal pay at the same level of employment, and these factors all impact health. Further examples include differential access to medical facilities (including proximity, physical access, financial access, and even linguistic access) and differential access to a clean environment (including the differential placement of toxic dump sites and the cynical designation of "sacrifice zones" near known polluting industries).

Examples of differences in access to power include differential access to information (including health information, as well as information about our own histories), differential access to resources (including both financial resources and social networking resources), and differential access to voice (including expressing one's voice in the media, in government, and through voting).

Observed associations between social class and "race" in this country do not "just so happen." They are the result of initial historical injustices that have been perpetuated by contemporary structural factors. That is, structural racism explains the association between social class and "race" in this country. Finally, structural racism can occur through acts of commission (doing) and through acts of omission (not doing). In fact, structural racism very often shows up these days as inaction in the face of need.

## On racism denial

Many people in the United States are in staunch denial that racism has ever existed in this country, that racism still exists in this country, and that racism continues to have profoundly negative impacts on the health and well-being of our whole nation. Racism denial is a huge "black hole" in our national landscape, massive and powerful. Recent manifestations of racism denial include the Supreme Court decision about affirmative action in higher education; efforts to suppress the teaching of our full American history by limiting discussions of American chattel slavery; and efforts to ban work on diversity, equity, and inclusion in government, educational institutions, and workplaces. Banned books, banned words, banned research, and banned speech are accelerating manifestations of racism denial as I write this foreword.

There are many axes of inequity operating in our society today, intersecting in communities and in individuals. These include race, gender, ethnicity, indigenous status, history of colonization, social class markers, relation to means of production, nationality, language, immigration status, sexual orientation, gender identity, gender expression, geography, age, religion, caste, disability status, weight status, incarceration history, substance use history, and mental health history.

So why focus our efforts and this book on "race" as the axis of inequity and on racism as the associated system of structured inequity? It is because racism is foundational in our nation's history and continues to have profoundly negative impacts on the health and well-being of our nation at the same time that racism denial is so staunchly held by so many in this country and is so seductive. This combination of racism being foundational and racism being denied makes me urge *all* of us to at least actively oppose racism, even as we also engage around as many of the other systems of structured inequity as we can manage. And to the extent that we are able to dismantle the mechanisms of racism, the other struggles will benefit as well.

## What can we do?

Antiracism is a process with three tasks: name racism, ask "How is racism operating here?" and organize and strategize to act.

1. We must *name racism*, say the whole word "race-ism," especially now with attacks on antiracism, diversity, equity, inclusion, belonging, justice, and equity. This can be difficult, but we must

name any problem to get started on the solution. However, as necessary as it is to name racism, it is also insufficient. We must go beyond naming racism and move to action.

2. Posing the question *"How is racism operating here?"* is the first step to action. We aim to identify the mechanisms of racism in the structures, policies, practices, norms, and values that are "here," within our setting and within our reach. This landscaping exercise helps us identify early targets for action and promising levers for intervention. Because this question lays the foundation for parts of the rest of this book, further details on how to answer this question are presented following this numbered list.
3. After identifying some of the mechanisms of racism in our setting and within our reach, we need to *organize and strategize to act.* I acknowledge that each of us has power to address racism as an individual. But collective action magnifies our individual power. Collective action informs us, inspires us, propels us, protects us, and so much more.

The three tasks of antiracism outlined above are sequential. In addition, the cycle of tasks will likely need to be repeated, again and again, as we confront racism denial while growing a cadre of antiracism activists. The fact that antiracism is a process that is sequential, iterative, and may well span generations should not discourage us. Antiracism is movement building, involving collective action, mobilization of a critical mass, intentional connections across generations, and persistence. We must be willing to start now and do our parts, even if we will not necessarily see the full and final win. We must be willing to plant acorns today so that our grandchildren will have shade.

## How is racism operating here?

To answer the question "How is racism operating here?" we need to examine the mechanisms of racism in our structures, policies, practices, norms, and values. Although this may seem daunting at first, we gain traction on this task when we recognize that structures, policies, practices, norms, and values are simply the elements of decision-making.

Structures are the "who," "what," "when," and "where" of decision-making. Who is at the decision-making table (and who is not)? What is on the agenda (and what is not)? At what times and in what settings are decisions made? Indeed, I strongly encourage every reader, whenever you find yourself at a decision-making table (or you set one), to ask yourself, "Who is *not* here who has an interest in this proceeding?" In recognizing who is *not* at the table, your job is to create space and find them a way to the table.

Policies are the *written* "how" of decision-making. How do the written rules of the game have the impact of differentially structuring opportunity by race? Note that no express intent is required. Just as with assessing who is not at the table and what is not on the agenda, it is very important to assess what policies are not in place that, if implemented, would result in more social justice. Indeed, seeing "the absence of" is a very important antiracism skill and orientation across many domains and activities.

Both practices and norms are the *unwritten* how of decision-making, differing mainly in their time scale and durability. Practices are the unwritten how, here and now. "Just watch me, you'll see how things are done!" Norms are the unwritten how that are deeply embedded in culture. They are clues as to whether a person belongs and are "the way we expect you to do things going forward."

Because practices and norms are unwritten, they are more difficult to discern when trying to answer the question, "How is racism operating here?" Norms are especially powerful, yet invisible, mechanisms of racism because they are rarely named, described, or interrogated. Indeed, rarely can an insider describe or identify a norm, while an outsider's flagging of a detrimental norm will usually be rejected as an attack on the group.

Finally, values are the "why" of decision-making. They govern the prioritization of populations, issues, approaches, and investments. They are manifest in differential rewards, attention, protection, investments, and invitation.

A quick rule of thumb about how to start intervening on decision-making processes to address racism: change who is at the decision-making table. That is because the who at the table also brings the what on the agenda, the problem identification and urgency for action. The who also brings the why, the relative weighing of competing priorities and the commitment or not to equity, to the assurance of the conditions for optimal health for all people. Indeed, the why includes who is even deemed worthy of consideration when resources are distributed and when limited resources require prioritization.

## Transforming Health Care: Creating Equitable, Antiracist Healthcare Organizations

I welcome you into acceptance of these four truths: that racism exists, that racism is a system, that racism saps the strength of the whole society, and that we can *all* act to dismantle racism. Please read on to know that this work is possible, impactful, and energizing. We have power, and when we work together, we can use that power to improve the health and well-being of those who have been dehumanized, marginalized, and overlooked—by doing so, we improve the health and well-being of all.

Camara Phyllis Jones, MD, PhD, MPH
Family Physician and Epidemiologist
Past President, American Public Health Association
Antiracism thought leader and activist
March 2025

## A Few Resources from Dr. Jones


1 Jones CP. Confronting institutionalized racism. *Phylon.* 2002; 50(1–2):7–22. https://doi.org/10.2307/4149999
2 Jones CP. Levels of racism: A theoretic framework and a gardener's tale. *Am J Public Health.* 2000; 90(8):1212–1215. PMCID: PMC1446334
3 Jones CP. Systems of power, axes of inequity: Parallels, intersections, braiding the strands. *Med Care.* 2014; 52(10 Suppl 3):S71–S75. https://doi.org/10.1097/MLR.0000000000000021
4 Jones CP, Jones CY, Jones CA. Anti-racism primer: Naming racism and moving to action. In: Holden KB, Jones CP, eds. *Black Women and Resilience: Power, Perseverance, and Public Health.* State University of New York Press; 2024: 365–388.
5 Jones CP, Truman BI, Elam-Evans LD, Jones CA, Jones CY, Jiles R, et al. Using "socially-assigned race" to probe White advantages in health status. *Ethn Dis.* 2008; 18(4):496–504; PMID:19157256

# Preface

Work on this book began early in 2024. As the manuscript was nearing completion, the 45th president of the United States was again sworn in as the 47th president of the United States. A large number of executive orders and other directives were immediately issued, and the new administration has continued to release an unprecedented torrent of communications from the executive branch on a large number of topics and issues. Federal websites, including many with important health-related informational and data resources, have been taken down. Rapid restructuring of federal agencies with massive layoffs/firings and immediate termination of long-standing programs and policies have already impacted many segments of the population and many sectors of the economy. The list of programs and policies affected by the recent executive orders will likely continue to grow, as will the uncertainty and anxiety generated by these actions. Each day brings new pronouncements from the executive branch about defunding various services for children, youth, adults, or seniors; services that the administration does not value; and declarations about new groups that will no longer be protected or will be actively prosecuted by federal officials.

As this manuscript is being submitted, less than three months after the inauguration, no laws have changed. There are (as yet) no "illegal words." Nevertheless, both individuals and organizations have begun acting on their uncertainty and unease by attempting to comply with the positions and policies being promulgated by the new administration. Some organizations are removing information from their websites about programs that are not aligned with the views of the new administration and circulating lists of what they think may be "illegal words." Individuals who belong to groups being targeted by the new administration have become fearful to travel, to visit public venues, or even to seek medical care as accounts are posted on social media about immigrants who are legal residents or even citizens of the United States who have been arbitrarily detained by the Immigration and Customs Enforcement (ICE) agency, and transgender persons who fear arrest for fraud if their passports have information that is discordant with the gender in which they are currently living.

Large public protests have already been organized across the country. Many of the new administration's actions have been challenged in court and some of their initiatives have been paused by injunctions, but it is clear that the administration will continue to pursue its agenda for the country. However, as all of this plays out over time, healthcare organizations must continue with their mission to provide high-quality care for all of their patients. For those who believe in science and who deal in facts, the reality of health disparities resulting from structural inequities must be addressed. Whatever words they may or may not use to describe their programs, healthcare leaders must continue to pursue strategies and initiatives to help obtain the best possible health outcomes for all of their patients. This book was written to support those efforts. We have included many online references and resources, some of which will no doubt be unavailable by the time this book is published. Nevertheless, we have endeavored to provide reliable and accurate information about the subject matter in each chapter to guide the work of becoming an antiracist healthcare organization.

Lynne D. Richardson, MD, and Sima Rabinowitz
March 30, 2025

# Acknowledgments

This book brings together—and owes a debt of gratitude to—the ideas, principles, and daily work of individuals, institutions, and organizations across the country who recognize that racial health equity is, indisputably, among the most important issues of our time. It is difficult to imagine any discussion of the ways in which racism operates in our society without the groundbreaking work of Dr. Camara Phyllis Jones, and we are honored that our book begins with her voice.

We are deeply grateful to Dr. Dennis S. Charney, former Dean of the Icahn School of Medicine at Mount Sinai, whose original suggestion was the impetus for this book.

We would like to express our profound appreciation to Kenneth L. Davis, MD, former Chief Executive Officer of the Mount Sinai Health System, and to the members of the Mount Sinai Health System Task Force to Address Racism and Discrimination (2020–2021), with special thanks to the Task Force Chair, Gary C. Butts, MD, and the members of the Task Force Strategy and Support team: Pamela Y. Abner, MPA, CPXP; Gabriel Bershadscky; Ben Cotilleta; Leona Hess, PhD, BS, MSW; Marc Kaplan; and Ann-Gel Palermo, DrPH, MPH, TIPC, ACC.

We have been inspired by and admire our colleagues at the Icahn School of Medicine at Mount Sinai and throughout the Mount Sinai Health System, who are champions of health equity, partners in the work, and deeply committed to the evolution of an equitable, antiracist health system, particularly Gary C. Butts, MD; Pamela Y. Abner, MBA, CPXP; Nina A. Bickell, MD, MPH; Yvette Calderon, MD, MS; Lyndia Hayden, MS, PMP; Doran Ricks, MS, RN, MBA; and Toni S. Stern, MD, MBA.

We recognize the invaluable work and support of Dr. Carol R. Horowitz and our many brilliant and extraordinary colleagues in the Institute for Health Equity Research at the Icahn School of Medicine at Mount Sinai. A special thank you goes to Eunice Wright for expert administrative support and to our talented independent researchers, Cordelia R. Elaiho, MPH; Dina Naphor, MA; and Allyson Riddle, MA.

We are grateful to the many healthcare leaders and innovators who graciously shared stories of their work with us and whose efforts are featured in the chapter Spotlights: Pamela Y. Abner, MBA, CPXP; Gary C. Butts, MD; Brendan G. Carr, MD, MA, MS; and Doran Ricks, MSN, RN, MBA, at the Mount Sinai Health System; Scott Cook, PhD; Mark Connolly, MEng; Mary Kate Selling, MHA; and James S. Williams Jr., MA, at UChicago Medicine; Lucy Marcil, MD, MPH, at Boston Medical Center; Nwamaka (Amaka) Eneanya, MD, MPH, at Emory Healthcare; Myra Gregorian, MA; Rosie Jones; Ian Johnson; Erin Murphy, MPS, MAIS; Wendy Price, MPA; and Alicia Tieder, MSW, LICSW, at Seattle Children's; Sean Brown, RN; Ann Gakumo, PhD, RN; Jordan Gayle, MBA; and Greer Glazer, RN, CNP, PhD, FANN, at the University of Cincinnati College of Nursing; John A. Rich, MD, MPH, from Rush University Medical Center; and Ayesha Jako, MAM, from West Side United.

Sarah Humphreville at Oxford University Press has championed this book from our earliest discussions in the spring of 2022 and has remained dedicated to the book's purpose through an unanticipated period of uncertainty and political change. We appreciate the labor involved in book production and wish to thank everyone at OUP for their efforts in bringing this volume to life.

Dr. Richardson would like to thank her daughters, Kristin Richardson Jordan and Lauren Richardson Jordan Newman, who bring her joy, make her proud, and give her hope.

Sima Rabinowitz would like to thank Lynne for inviting her to embark on this journey and the opportunity to think deeply about the ideas and practices we have explored together here, and Susan Denelsbeck, for accompanying her on so many challenging journeys over more than three decades and counting.

# Table Caption/Credit List



This table presents select, representative examples of action plan recommendations. This is not a comprehensive or exhaustive list.



Adapted from multiple sources on SODH and social needs screening tools:

Center for Health Equity Advancement. Health Disparities and Social Determinants of Health. University of Pennsylvania. Philadelphia, PA. https://www.chea.upenn.edu/health-disparities-and-social-determinants-of-health/

Healthy People 2030, U.S. Department of Health and Human Services, Office of Disease Prevention and Health Promotion. Social Determinants of Health. https://odphp.health.gov/healthypeople/objectives-and-data/social-determinants-health

National Association of Community Health Centers, Inc., Association of Asian Pacific Community Health Organizations, and Oregon Primary Care Association. 2016. The PRAPRE® Screening Tool. https://prapare.org/the-prapare-screening-tool/

Social Interventions Research and Evaluations Network (siren). Social Needs Screening Tool Comparison Table. University of California, San Francisco. 2019. September 2024. https://sirenetwork.ucsf.edu/tools-resources/resources/screening-tools-comparison

# Introduction

Elimination of the pervasive and persistent racial/ethnic disparities in life expectancy, disease burden, and health outcomes has been a national public health goal in the United States for more than 30 years. Despite substantial progress, Black, Latine, Native American, and other racial/ethnic population groups continue to experience poorer health. The causes of these disparities are multifactorial and are deeply influenced by adverse social determinants at the individual level (lack of education, poverty) and the neighborhood level (environmental toxins, community disinvestment). It is now well understood that racism, bias, and discrimination contribute substantially to these disparate health outcomes.

## Note on Terminology

There is ongoing conversation among advocates and academics regarding the appropriate term for individuals who are currently (and historically) classified by the federal government as Hispanic, a term used by some members of this group to refer to themselves, but one that was never embraced by many others, and which describes a language affiliation (people of Spanish-speaking ancestry). Latino (male) and Latina (female) are terms used to describe individuals, and the male form, Latino, has been widely used for the past 50 or 60 years when referring to this group of people, both by those who are members of the group and by those who are not. Over the past two decades, those seeking a nongendered term to describe the group have adopted the term Latinx, which was coined in the early 2000s. This term has met with

*continued*

*Transforming Health Care*. Lynne D. Richardson and Sima Rabinowitz, Oxford University Press.
 DOI: 10.1093/oso/9780197805374.003.0001

*continued*

some resistance in the community because "x" (when pronounced "ex") is not a sound that occurs in the Spanish language. In this book, we will use the term Latine (pronounced *lat-in-ay*), which has recently emerged as a gender-neutral term in the English language to refer to this expansive ethnic group of individuals with ancestry in North, Central, and South America and the Caribbean and who represent an enormous diversity of languages (Spanish, Portuguese, indigenous languages) and cultures.

In early 2020, the devastating impact of the COVID-19 pandemic on Black and Latine communities was highlighted in both traditional and social media, raising awareness of the preexisting, long-standing inequities that contributed to the staggering death toll from SARS CoV-2 in urban Black communities early in the pandemic. However, it was public outrage over the televised murder of George Floyd by a White police officer that sparked an unprecedented reaction across the United States as Americans experienced a collective epiphany—a striking realization that anti-Black racism is part of the current lived experience in this country. Individuals from all backgrounds, including the leadership of corporations, institutions, and organizations from every sector, began to recognize that they had been complacent, if not complicit, in perpetuating systemic racism. Public declarations and position statements decrying racism and espousing the elimination of bias, discrimination, and inequitable treatment abounded.

More than 260 municipalities across the United States have declared racism a public health crisis.[1] In 2021, the Centers for Disease Control and Prevention (CDC) issued the same declaration,[2] the National Institutes of Health (NIH)[3] named structural racism as a priority, and the American Medical Association(AMA)[4] announced a plan to embed racial justice within its organization. Many organizations and companies across many sectors and industries have, over the past two or three years, published components of their strategic plans to address racism and advance equity on their websites. Educational organizations have been particularly active, with many of them adding antiracist themes and content to their curricula.

Many healthcare organizations that are sites for the education and training of physicians, nurses, nurse practitioners, physician assistants, social workers, and allied health personnel have witnessed this trend in their affiliated health professions schools. Significant scholarship has demonstrated that race is a social category that reflects the impact of unequal social experiences on health and dispelled the myth that race is a biologic category based on innate differences. Most U.S. medical schools launched antiracism initiatives to help students, as well as faculty and staff, understand how racism functions in our society and how it affects patients, colleagues, organizations, and workplaces.

Educational sessions focus on understanding the relationships among race, racism, and health; the cultural, social, and historical context of the structural inequities that drive many of the disparities that exist; and the impact of racial bias in research, clinical practice, and medical education. Medical school courses now routinely incorporate topics such as unconscious bias, microaggressions, allyship, consideration of self-identity and privilege, and recognition of oppressive and racism-sustaining organizational behaviors. Training modules for students, faculty, and staff help learners develop awareness of individual biases, including implicit bias, and teach skills for bystander intervention, de-escalation, and conflict resolution to address the harms that racism creates. Curricula also delve into the intersections of social determinants of health and healthcare disparities, helping students understand the multifaceted barriers to health and health care, and teach cultural competency skills in caring for patients from diverse backgrounds, including all racial, ethnic, religious, and cultural groups, as well as individuals who identify as lesbian, gay, bisexual, transgender, nonbinary, queer, or questioning (LGBTQ).

Nursing professional societies and schools offer a similarly robust variety of antiracism tools, trainings, and resources on their websites. These offerings are designed to describe the impact of racism on patients and nurses; improve skills and provide encouragement to confront individual and systemic racism; promote culturally appropriate models of effective nursing care; and stimulate innovation and problem-solving to address these disparities and inequities. Many identify antiracist teaching and learning resources (brief lectures and case-based learning) and measurement tools for nurse educators; some describe strategies to address racism in academic clinical settings. Other initiatives focus on increasing diversity in the nursing workforce through pipeline and mentorship programs, scholarships, and leadership development programs. Similar initiatives have been launched in other health disciplines, including social work, physical therapy, psychology, midwifery education, and public health.

Healthcare leaders, like their counterparts in education, must acknowledge that the existing inequalities in health and health outcomes stem from structural racism and the macrolevel bias intrinsic in the design and operations of healthcare institutions, as well as implicit bias among clinicians and other staff. This book is designed to guide and support healthcare organizations that are committed to the goal of becoming equitable, antiracist organizations.

Although much of the conversation about race in America is centered on anti-Black racism, we recognize that bias and discrimination are experienced based on many characteristics, including race, ethnicity, sexual orientation, gender identity, disability status, nationality, immigration status, housing status, former incarceration, religion, medical diagnosis, behavioral diagnosis, education, and occupation. The lived experiences of each group are unique, but both the antecedents and the consequences of inequity are similar across groups. Individuals who experience bias and discrimination may endure direct adverse health effects and face structural barriers to accessing the resources needed to attain and maintain health; some may be heirs of historical disadvantage and generational trauma. Many individuals have intersecting identities that confer multiple adverse health impacts. The strategies described in this book can be used to advance health equity for all marginalized and disadvantaged populations.

It is essential that those who seek to transform health care into an equitable system that values everyone and provides high-quality care to all understand the myriad, insidious ways in which policies and practices rooted in racism are entrenched throughout society and, more specifically, how such policies and practices are embedded throughout health care. We must learn to look at every aspect of the enterprise and ask ourselves: "How is racism operating here?" We must learn to look beneath the surface, to question underlying assumptions, and to question dogma. It is a lengthy, sometimes painful, always challenging process. In this book, we will share the knowledge of individuals who have thought deeply about these issues and the experiences of organizations that have already embarked on this journey.

## Organization of This Book

In Chapter 1, we describe how to design and implement a comprehensive process to achieve transformational change in a healthcare organization. This type of change must be supported at the highest level of the organization—be it a single hospital or a clinic or a large healthcare system. We discuss the methods and tools required, including communications mechanisms and leadership training models. We also describe the importance of choosing an evaluation framework to monitor progress. Undertaking this type of holistic change requires thoughtful planning, a substantial organizational investment of resources, and a sustained commitment to do the hard work required to examine and modify structures, policies, practices, norms, and values throughout the organization.

In Chapters 2, 3, and 4, we consider the ways in which structural inequities manifest themselves in the clinical arena, how racism is embedded in the delivery of clinical care, and how to detect and eliminate interpersonal racism in clinical encounters. Key strategies to be employed include embedding equity into the measurement of care quality throughout the organization, committing to ensuring equitable access to clinical services, and achieving equitable patient outcomes across all racial, ethnic, and language groups. The role of healthcare organizations in screening for and addressing health-related social needs is described, as well as their responsibility to eliminate discriminatory practices, policies, and clinical tools and to establish and maintain a bias-free environment both for patients and their families and for staff.

In Chapter 5, we describe how to eliminate both overt and structural racism from business structures, processes, and practices, both externally and internally. Internally, this involves a detailed examination of existing human resources systems and processes, including pay equity analyses; development of recruitment, hiring, and retention practices that promote diversity and equity; creating professional and leadership development opportunities, mentorship and sponsorship programs and workforce training and development programs; and careful assessment of evaluation and promotion criteria and processes to eliminate bias and discrimination. Externally, this requires implementation of strategies for diversifying the supply chain and for leveraging purchasing power and investments in real estate, facilities, and equipment to promote local small businesses and provide workforce development opportunities in local communities.

In Chapter 6, we address the need for continuous learning and leadership to sustain the process of change. We discuss leveraging in-house and outside expertise and describe the design, delivery, and evaluation of tailored training programs and resources for executives and staff at all levels. Chapter 7 focuses on the importance of multi-sector partnerships and adopting an anchor mission in creating and sustaining change. Collaborating with community stakeholders, organizations, and institutions is essential to the change process and to the development of thriving local economies; the voices of the communities being served must be at the table to help redesign care processes to achieve equitable outcomes. Healthcare organizations must work more closely with public health professionals to eliminate environmental inequities that threaten health. Healthcare organizations also have a key role to play in partnering with payors, policy makers, elected officials, and regulators to eliminate barriers to sustainable change.

This book provides ways to consider creating sustained, transformative organizational change. It may be that some organizations have embarked on the process of change and have already accomplished some of the work described. We also recognize that not all organizations are ready to undertake comprehensive change or have the resources available to initiate sweeping change. We have organized the book so that individual chapters can be used to address specific aspects of a healthcare organization. We encourage readers to use the book in the way that best serves them.

## Spotlight Stories

The book also includes seven brief "Spotlight" stories highlighting antiracism and racial health equity initiatives of health and hospital systems and healthcare leaders across the country. These stories describe an organization's antiracism action plan (Chapter 1); development and implementation of a quality metrics scorecard to identify healthcare disparities (Chapter 2); a medical–financial partnership in a pediatric clinic (Chapter 3); implementation of a race-neutral clinical algorithm and equity transformation initiatives (Chapter 4); antiracist human resources practices (Chapter 5); an antiracism nursing school curriculum collaborative (Chapter 6); and a successful health anchor initiative (Chapter 7).

## The Future of Diversity, Equity, and Inclusion

As we write this book, initiatives to support diversity, equity, and inclusion are under attack across the country by forces that are interested in maintaining the advantaged position of White people in our society. Laws that ban diversity initiatives in various venues have been enacted in many states, and federal legislation has been introduced. Whatever the outcome of these efforts, we believe that the moral imperative and practical rationale for dismantling racism in America will continue to motivate healthcare organizations to transform themselves into antiracist organizations. From an ethical perspective, perpetuation of a system that disadvantages people based on how they look is at odds with the principles that guide health professionals: autonomy (respect for each person's right to make decisions), beneficence (the duty to "do good"), nonmaleficence (the duty to do no harm), and justice (the duty to treat all people equitably). From a business point of view, healthcare organizations, like other businesses, recognize both the changing demographics of the United States and the performance advantage of diverse teams.

Transforming a healthcare organization into a diverse, equitable, antiracist workplace is the smart thing to do. Providing high-quality, equitable health care, regardless of a patient's background or identity, is the right thing to do. In this book, we describe the issues to be considered, the resources needed, and the strategies to be implemented as healthcare organizations embark on, or in some cases continue, this journey of transformation.

## References

1. Lapeyrouse LM, Key KD, Bailey S. Operationalizing racism as a public health crisis: Moving beyond the rhetoric! *J Particip Res Methods.* 2024; 5(2). https://doi.org/10.35844/001c.120289
2. Centers for Disease Control and Prevention. Media Release from Director Rochelle P. Wolensky, MD, MPH, on Racism and Health. Accessed February 10, 2025. https://archive.cdc.gov/www_cdc_gov/media/releases/2021/s0408-racism-health.html
3. Collins FS, Adams AB, Aklin C, Archer TK, Bernard MA, Boone E, Burklow J, et al. Affirming NIH's commitment to addressing structural racism in the biomedical research enterprise. *Cell.* 2021 Jun 10; 184(12):3075–3079. https://doi.org/10.1016/j.cell.2021.05.014
4. O'Reilley KB. Health equity. Racism is a threat to public health. American Medical Association. November 16, 2020. https://www.ama-assn.org/delivering-care/health-equity/ama-racism-threat-public-health

# 1

# How Is Racism Operating Here?

## Developing an Antiracism Action Plan

Do the images on signs and posters throughout the hospital and in clinic waiting rooms depict only White patients? Are telehealth appointments offered to some patients, but not to others with similar health conditions? Would an analysis of patient medical records show a difference in the way clinicians routinely describe the behaviors or self-reported symptoms of Black and White patients? Do hospital readmission rates differ for patient groups by race or ethnicity? Has a Black physician ever been stopped in the hospital corridors by a security guard and asked to show identification? Does the health system's workforce reflect the diversity of the communities it serves? Do the hospital's vendors include local minority-owned businesses?

When we ask the question *How is racism operating here?*, these are the types of scenarios we are thinking about, among many others, and the sorts of questions we should be asking. How are inequitable, unjust, discriminatory, or biased practices and policies impacting our employees, our patients, and the larger community in both pervasive and specific ways? We must examine how racism is embedded in our institutional practices and policies and how they contribute to disparities in health outcomes, in patient experience, and in engagement with our communities.

How do we uncover these problems, begin to address them, and transform the underlying structures and systems that perpetuate them? In this chapter, we will describe the development of organizational structures and system-wide plans, strategies, and activities designed to operationalize an antiracist vision and rigorously evaluate progress toward achieving it.

*Transforming Health Care*. Lynne D. Richardson and Sima Rabinowitz, Oxford University Press.
 DOI: 10.1093/oso/9780197805374.003.0002

## Establishing Antiracism as a Core Value and Strategic Priority

The first, and a fundamentally important, step is establishing racial equity as a core organizational value and the work of actively dismantling racism as a strategic priority. To move with purpose and intention toward this goal, it is critical to disrupt what has been called "race silence,"[1] or an unwillingness to talk openly and explicitly about racism, by naming it and recognizing past harms. Organizational leaders must acknowledge that racism and inequities exist and operate throughout society, including in our own organizations, and must demonstrate a public commitment to antiracism.

Although many organizations across the country have publicly identified health equity as a core value or organizational priority, for example, with statements on their websites and in patient-facing materials, it will be impossible to achieve health equity without also striving for racial equity. An explicit commitment to dismantling racism demonstrates awareness of this work as an organizational imperative that is an essential component of health equity.

A coordinated effort to assess and redress racism is a complex undertaking that, in every organization, regardless of size, will require critical resources—a significant investment of time, personnel, a dedicated budget—and the establishment of formal organizational structures and system-wide plans. Executive leaders should engage experts (internal professionals and/or external consultants) with deep expertise in racial equity and justice work to join them in establishing a formal process of advancing antiracism, beginning with the articulation of racial equity as a core value. This should include appointing a senior executive–level individual to lead this work, for example, a chief health equity officer, who will report directly to the organization's chief executive officer or president and be accountable, as relevant, to other governing groups, such as a board of trustees.

### Transparency and Accountability

To ensure that the value statement is not merely performative, but also authentic and actionable, dismantling racism must also become a strategic organizational priority—in other words, a measurable, time-bound set of goals and objectives with clear targets and metrics. Given that anti-Black racism and White privilege have been normalized and are often therefore (and mistakenly) understood to be absent, transparency and accountability are especially critical. An organization's executive and senior leaders must be held accountable not only for their own performance, but also for organizational performance when it comes to implementing and sustaining antiracist practices and policies. Some organizations, for example, have tied achievement of specific antiracism goals and objectives to executive compensation. Others have required leaders to participate in mandatory, ongoing training and development to help ensure that they are prepared to lead and sustain antiracism efforts.

Accountability is ideally accompanied by transparency. Leaders must not only announce their values, intentions, and plans for the organization (and for themselves), but also engage individuals at all levels in the work of dismantling racism and communicate openly and often about antiracism initiatives. We will return to these themes (leadership development, engagement, and communication) later in this chapter.

Dismantling racism as an organizational imperative involves changing beliefs and behaviors, culture and climate, and practices and policies across every level and function of the organization from boardroom to bedside, human resources to research lab, health records to vendor contracts, and medical education curricula to patient intake procedures. Once antiracism has been articulated as a strategic priority, the next critical step is to bring people from throughout the organization together to develop a formal plan for change.

## Creating an Antiracism Action Plan: Processes to Support Change

A number of healthcare organizations, primarily large academic medical centers, have developed and shared comprehensive and detailed antiracism or racial equity plans (typically called action plans or road maps) to guide assessment of their existing state (processes, policies, practices, programs, workplace culture, etc.) and to develop specific recommendations for moving the organization forward to create a more just, antiracist, and equitable organization.[2–5] A large number of state governments, nonprofit organizations, and health-care foundations have published handbooks, manuals, and toolkits to help guide large-scale institutional change to advance health and racial equity, which are freely available online.[6,7] We have included several of these in our Recommended Reading and Resources at the end of the chapter.

Although antiracism action plans or road maps differ based on the size and characteristics of the institutions, among other factors, organizations that are engaged in large-scale change initiatives share a set of common overarching processes and key components, which typically include:

- establishment of a formal organizational structure to carry out the work (a "change management team" with administrative support and dedicated resources);
- definition of core domains for change (a set of key themes, pillars, or major strategic areas);
- creation of a realistic timeline for *development* of the action plan, with a timeline for *implementation* of the plan's recommendations to follow (a detailed outline of milestones and deadlines);
- identification of processes and methods for an organizational self-assessment and collection and review of data (quantitative and qualitative information and perspectives);
- development of explicit recommendations, proposed actions, or interventions for each domain, theme, or area (measurable goals to be achieved);
- creation of an implementation and governance plan (*what, when, where, how, who*); and
- adoption or design of an evaluation framework (metrics, accountability).

Plans for large-scale organizational change are, by their nature, ambitious. Yet, by ambitious we do not mean aspirational. To be effective, health and racial equity action plans must also be robust and durable, reflecting a highly coordinated effort with the inclusion of explicit goals and tactics.

## Organization-Wide Coalitions

It seems fair to say that the change team—whether defined as a task force, planning committee, or coalition—will be one of the largest groups an organization has ever assembled focused on a unified goal. Given the imperative to effect change at every level of the organization, it is important to involve people from throughout the organization to serve in this group. It should include both individuals who have previously led or engaged in antiracism work and those who have not and should reflect a range of expertise, experience, perspectives, rank, and personal characteristics (race, ethnicity, age, gender or gender identity, ability/disability). It is helpful to engage those who have experience in prior antiracism work, or other relevant experience, to serve on an executive steering committee or another lead entity to guide the overall process and to help ensure accountability.

Organization-wide coalitions can include members from corporate service and operations units (business, finance, human resources, public affairs and media, and patient experience officers and staff); clinical and nonclinical hospital staff (physicians, nurses, residents, lab technicians, registrars, allied health professionals, hospital cafeteria workers); medical and nonmedical clinic staff (physicians, medical assistants, nurse practitioners, front-desk staff); academic departments (deans, chairs, faculty members, students, alumni); special offices (community affairs); and trustees or board members. To engage expertise or perspectives that are not represented on the task force, organizations could consider engaging additional "field experts" or "internal consultants" throughout the organization over the course of its work to provide feedback as plans are developed. Organizations should include patients and local community leaders on these coalitions or on associated subcommittees or work groups, which strengthens the work and provides an opportunity to build or enhance community engagement.

If there are earlier, ongoing, or parallel efforts in place within the institution, such as departmental antiracism initiatives, related employee affinity or resource groups, or curriculum projects in health professions training programs, it is important to bring people who are involved in such work into the lager antiracism action plan process. These individuals will have valuable expertise and institutional knowledge to help advance a unified vision while reducing the chances of duplicating effort and missing opportunities for synergies.

Dedicated administrative support is critical for success if development of an antiracism action plan is to remain a priority, including a team to manage logistics (coordinating meeting schedules, setting up and maintaining document management and sharing systems, etc.), ensure continuity, and help sustain the effort over time. It may be necessary to hire staff or to adjust roles to ensure sufficient staffing for this important work without overburdening existing staff. As the project develops, additional support may be necessary to operationalize the plan, for example, data analysts to review and interpret the data that will drive the development and implementation of specific recommendations or interventions. The administrative support team will want to work closely with the executive steering committee to select a project management strategy, develop mechanisms for sharing materials, document the process, and create a system for tracking progress across the various phases of creating and implementing the action plan.

It is likely that most healthcare leaders will not have previously been involved in orchestrating large antiracism efforts and may wish or need to engage outside consultants. Professional racial justice and equity consulting firms, several of which specialize in health care, can assist with the development of core values statements, environmental scans and self-assessment, implementation of participatory processes to guide the coalition in consensus building and equitable decision-making processes, selection and adaptation of evaluation frameworks, and developing and conducting antiracism leadership training.

## Frameworks for Change

As we have said, advancing this work with a large coalition and the imperative to create an actionable, measurable set of recommendations or interventions is no small undertaking. It may be helpful to adopt a formal organizational or social change methodology to help guide the process, which can be led by internal experts, outside consultants, or a combination of internal and external experts.[8–10] At the very least, it will be essential to put in place a process for participatory (equitable) decision-making—in other words, a method and mechanisms for sharing opinions, encouraging and engaging in small- and large-group dialogue, and testing for consensus before finalizing decisions.[10]

It is helpful to remember that the purpose of the organizational task force or coalition is to determine *whether* and *why* a change is necessary (where racist or discriminatory processes or practices are operating), *what* the goals and outcomes of the change should be, and *how* these goals can be achieved. The group charged with this critical endeavor must embody and model equity principles by continuing to apply a racial justice lens to its own work by asking: *Who is not in the room with us who should be? Who benefits from the decisions we make, and who may be harmed by them?*

## Creating an Antiracism Action Plan: Recommendations, Interventions, Implementation, and Evaluation

Large health and hospital systems and academic medical centers have typically designed their antiracism action plans around one of three organizing schemes. One is to define a small set of core, people-centric priority areas or pillars, for example, personnel (leaders and employees), patient care (patients and their families), and the broader community (multisector partnerships, public health or health policy initiatives).[2,7] The second is to define a limited set of overarching theme areas or categories ("healthcare delivery"; "learning and enrichment"; "clinical care").[3,4] The third is to identify a set of key themes or strategies that are framed as statements or as imperatives ("eliminate use of racially biased algorithms and tools"; "address social determinants of health"; "include patients in antiracism and health equity efforts").[5,11,12] Regardless of the action plan scheme, whether it includes these three or any other, the underlying principle is for the plan to encompass every aspect of the organization on some level: what it does, how it does it, with whom, and for whom.

## Data Collection and Review

Once key areas or themes have been defined, a common approach has been for subcommittees or work groups of the larger task force to engage in data collection and review from which to develop specific recommendations and interventions. Work groups often include members from throughout the organization who have not been involved in the larger task force coalition but who bring additional expertise or perspectives to the conversation.

Data collection to assess current practices, policies, programs, and perspectives might take the form of surveys and interviews, listening tours and town halls, review of existing materials and practices, and investigation of published reports and literature from other organizations. One option is to adapt an existing racial equity organizational self-assessment tool to help guide the collection of relevant data and information, which can be used with individuals and/or groups both to collect information and as a way to engage people in dialogue about themes and issues.[7,13,14] Depending on the size of the organization and the volume and complexity of the data, it may be helpful or necessary to hire data analysts specifically for this phase of the work or to realign current roles to ensure that the work can be done well and in a timely manner without overburdening staff. For this process to be effective, it is critical to be clear and transparent about accountability: who is ultimately responsible for overseeing the work and delivering the results?

Based on the collection, review, and interpretation of data from all levels of the organization, priority areas or key themes and strategies are then further broken down into more focused goals or objectives, accompanied by specific action steps and associated metrics (as we will describe next). Developing these steps may involve expanding or reforming the work groups, and, once again, engaging others in the organization and/or community members whose expertise or experience may be important or necessary to accomplish this work. Table 1.1 presents examples of broad organizational areas or categories that might be included in an action plan, with examples of associated recommendations or interventions and sample action steps.

**Table 1.1** Examples of Antiracism Action Plan Recommendations.

| Category | Recommendation |
|---|---|
| Infrastructure | Develop an organizational equity scorecard<br>Design an investment plan to support action plan recommendations<br>Create an organization-wide communications plan |
| Organizational culture | Require antiracism training for all leaders and managers<br>Implement a racism and discrimination reporting system<br>Disseminate antiracism learning and training resources |
| Clinical care | Review all clinical algorithms and calculators and eliminate any biased algorithms that inappropriately use race<br>Incorporate self-reported data on social determinants into each patient's electronic health record<br>Increase and improve language interpreter services |
| Workforce | Assess challenges for recruitment, hiring, and retention of employees from all backgrounds<br>Develop focused career advancement and mentorship programs<br>Conduct a pay equity analysis |
| Community | Establish relationships with local minority-owned and women-owned businesses<br>Engage patients and community stakeholders in the design of strategies to increase access to care<br>Partner with local community-based organizations to address health-related social needs |

*Note*: This table presents select, representative examples of action plan recommendations. This is not a comprehensive or exhaustive list.

## Metrics and Measurement

An antiracism action plan is intended to guide changes in organizational culture, practices, and policies and will encompass an expansive set of interventions and activities across widely different domains and functions, areas that are not typically assessed as part of a unified effort. Many experts recommend identifying a common set of performance indicators or measures, or what is called a shared measurement system, that will reflect shared goals and priorities across the entire organization.[8,15] Briefly, the purpose of a shared measurement system is to align what will be measured and how, along with methods and mechanisms for monitoring progress toward achieving goals; create benchmarks to help ensure accountability; share learning; and use this shared learning to inform strategies for change, improvement, and refinement or for determining new or additional metrics.

Not surprisingly, measurement proves to be a significant challenge for many organizations, with abstract targets and lack of training being key barriers to success.[16] Although designing and implementing metrics and a system of measurement may require a significant investment of time and resources, this step will be critical to the action plan's success. Ultimately, the goal of shared measurement is to support transparent, evidence-based decision-making to ensure transformative processes and outcomes and create sustainable change.

## Implementing the Action Plan

To be ready for implementation, an action plan or road map should comprise a set of goals and objectives and should describe the following for each goal or objective: (1) the purpose or rationale, which includes an assessment of current challenges or barriers; (2) the accountable leaders and responsible individuals; (3) a set of specific actions to be taken; (4) a set of metrics for each action, with milestones or measures of success for each action; and (5) resources needed (such as infrastructure, data collection, expertise in a specific area) and additional information about processes or methods for achieving results, informational sources, or alignment with other goals.

The final plan will reflect the input of individuals and teams from throughout the organization. To integrate enterprise-wide efforts, organizations will want to develop a governance model for the action plan with clearly delineated top-down (investment, advocacy) and bottom-up (input, implementation) responsibilities with detailed descriptions of goals and roles, expectations, and timelines.

## Designing an Evaluation Framework

As with any change effort, large or small, assessing the effectiveness and impact of the interventions is fundamental to understanding both what has worked and what has not; careful evaluation is needed to inform decision-making, continuous improvement, and sustainability. Evaluation is a complex process, and selection or adaptation of an appropriate theory or framework will ensure a holistic assessment that is relevant and impactful. Engaging a combination of internal and external experts and stakeholders may be especially useful in the selection or adaptation of an evaluation framework and development of progress reports.

Given the action plan's scope, namely, the intention to impact the whole of the organization in achieving racial equity, evaluation will likely involve combining and integrating the results of a vast set of success metrics that have been collected to assess the impact on organizational goals (operational, financial, clinical, etc.). The evaluation framework should enable stakeholders throughout the organization, as well as community partners, to understand the specific tangible outcomes of the action plan's implementation. *What has changed? How? Who has benefited, and how? What work remains to be accomplished? How will the changes be sustained?*

## **Engaging and Communicating**

The action plan's effectiveness will depend, at least in part, on conveying the message that the work of dismantling racism is the responsibility of every individual in the organization.[17] It will be important to devote sufficient time and resources to creating a well-orchestrated communications plan to promote awareness and engagement. Many organizations opt to include a representative from the organization's marketing and communications team to serve on the task force or coalition's executive steering committee. A communications work group can support the development of messages and materials in collaboration with individuals throughout the organization. In whatever ways the work is structured, formal communications and engagement strategies are key at every phase, from articulation of antiracism as a core value and establishment of the broad antiracism task force or coalition, to the collection of data that will inform the action plan, to the development and implementation of proposed recommendations and interventions, to evaluation.

Engagement strategies may include surveys to assess employees' perceptions and experiences; town halls to introduce plans and solicit feedback; tailored listening tours to engage in dialogue with departments, units, or teams; customized presentations delivered to leaders, managers, and boards; or special events (movies, guest speakers, action plan summits). Book clubs, conducted virtually or in person, centered on racial equity themes and intended for staff at all levels (with free access to the print volume or e-book to be discussed) provide an opportunity for employees who might not otherwise have the chance to interact with each other to come together to explore antiracist ideas. Similarly, "conversations" or "chats" centered on specific topics (racism in patient care; unconscious bias in the health-care workplace) led by antiracism experts can support action plan goals.

Communications activities, channels, and mechanisms could include:

- a dedicated antiracism action plan website with links to fact sheets, progress reports, videos, etc.;
- town hall meetings conducted centrally or at various sites or units throughout the organization and for all shifts (day, evening, night, weekends);
- presentations and question-and-answer sessions conducted in divisions, departments, or units;

- regular e-bulletins (weekly, monthly, or quarterly) or newsletters presenting key themes and highlighting progress (these should be archived on the action plan website);
- videos featuring leaders, task force members, and employees engaged in antiracism work throughout the organization, distributed electronically, presented in meetings or town halls, and archived on the action plan website;
- electronic bulletin boards posted at locations throughout the organization;
- news releases; and
- action plan or road map toolkits and training resources.

As an organizational value, equity must drive engagement and communications. This means ensuring that employees at all levels, wherever they work in the organization and whatever their role, must be included in, and have access to, engagement opportunities and communications. Events should be scheduled to optimize participation. Electronic newsletters or bulletins can be designed for easy viewing on mobile devices and surveys can be created for distribution on mobile devices. An option to encourage and facilitate engagement is the creation of designated computer workstation areas (for example, in staff lounges) where employees who do not have daily access to computers as a part of their work can participate in surveys or in online antiracism training activities.[14]

It is helpful to track engagement to ensure that all parts of the organization are being reached. Examples include monitoring "open rates" for e-bulletins or newsletters, uptake of hard-copy documents distributed around the organization, and attendance figures at town halls and other events. Interactive formats that include feedback mechanisms and options for employees to suggest topics for newsletters can enhance engagement and will provide key information to inform the action plan and antiracism efforts.

## Enhancing Leadership

Antiracism will be a new concept for many leaders. The work to actively dismantle racism may require new ways of thinking, as well as training to enhance knowledge and antiracism competencies. Experienced internal and/or external experts in antiracism can help leaders build capacity to recognize how racism manifests within the organization and apply a racial equity framework. Longitudinal training to support skill development over time is likely to be more effective than one-time sessions.[18]

Leadership training can be tailored to specific groups (executives, senior leaders responsible for development and implementation of the action plan, board members) and might combine self-assessment exercises, workshops, individual coaching, small- or large-group activities, videos, and a variety of evaluation materials. Antiracism training typically incorporates opportunities for self-reflection—an exploration of one's own racial identity, among other themes—learning about structural and systemic racism, and opportunities to cultivate the skills needed to advance the organization's antiracist objectives. Chapter 6 presents a more in-depth discussion of antiracist leadership models and practices.

## Summary

1. Examine how racism is embedded in internal institutional practices and policies. It will be impossible to achieve health equity without also striving for racial equity.
2. Engage individuals from throughout the organization, as well as internal and external experts, in antiracism work to develop a formal, organization-wide action plan or road map.
3. Organize the action plan around large key themes or strategies, followed by data collection, analysis of findings, and the subsequent breakdown of these larger themes into more focused, measurable objectives or goals.
4. Design and implement a system of metrics and milestones and an appropriate evaluation framework.
5. Implement communication and engagement strategies to engage people at every level of the organization and along every phase of the antiracism journey.

## SPOTLIGHT

### Road Map for Action to Address Racism

*Charging the health system's top leaders with sharing accountabilities and implementing the key strategies within their own areas of responsibility was an essential element of the Road Map.*

Dr. Gary Butts, MD, Executive Vice President for Diversity and Chief Diversity and Inclusion Officer for the Mount Sinai Health System; Dean for Diversity Programs, Policy, and Community Affairs for the Icahn School of Medicine at Mount Sinai; and Chair of the Task Force

In 2020, the intersecting public health crises of COVID-19 and racism drove a sense of urgency to unify and systematize antiracism efforts for leaders of the Mount Sinai Health System, one of the largest academic medical centers in New York City. Aiming to develop a comprehensive plan for system-wide commitment to becoming an antiracist, fair, and equitable community for its staff, patients, and students, the Chief Executive Officer (2003–2023), Dr. Kenneth Davis, convened a Task Force of 51 members, including a 5-member strategy and support team, from all levels throughout the organization. Task Force members represented corporate services units, health system hospitals, ambulatory clinics, academic departments, and the board of trustees. This work was grounded in a set of guiding principles that reflected the institution's core values and centered racial and social justice, encouraged task force members (and everyone throughout the organization) to name and speak up about racism, required a commitment to rebalancing power, and demanded both accountability and sustained commitment for the long term. The Task Force produced a *Road Map for Action to Address Racism*, which was designed to guide the organization's work.

The Road Map outlined a set of key strategies, and senior institutional leaders (chief clinical officer, chief financial officer, senior vice presidents, senior deans, and others) were charged with overseeing further development and implementation of each strategy. The Task Force concluded its work and was dissolved, as planned, after about 18 months. Strategy leads continued the work of implementing, evolving, and evaluating the Road Map, including a rigorous process of comprehensive data collection (clinical metrics, assessment of community partnerships, evaluation of investment plans, review of human resources strategies, etc.) and the design of governance structures and interventions for change.

Measuring and sharing metrics and system-wide performance was an important component of the Road Map. Process and outcomes measures for each strategy have been disseminated, as they become available, through a periodic e-bulletin sent to all 42,000+ health system employees, as well as through annual reports published on the health system's website. Road Map interventions included, among many other things, professional development and specialized mentoring programs seeking to accelerate career growth; a directed supply chain program; a locally focused nursing internship initiative; new policies and training to guide employees in responding to racist patient behavior; and the Health Equity Data Assessment (HEDA) Hub Portal, which hosted equity dashboards and a social determinants of health data collection tool, among many other Road Map efforts. "The HEDA Hub is a resource that allows us to engage our health system in data-driven equity initiatives and catalyze efforts to measure and monitor progress towards the provision of equitable health care," says Pamela Abner, MBA, CPXP, Senior Vice President, Chief Diversity Operations Officer, and Chief Health Equity Officer for the Mount Sinai Health System. According to Brendan Carr, MD, the current Chief Executive Officer of the Mount Sinai Health System, "the Road Map was an effective tool for aligning strategy with data driven benchmarks as we ensure equitable care to the communities that trust us with their lives."

In 2023, Mount Sinai joined the national Racial Health Equity Progress Report initiative, which is led by a collaboration of health equity, evaluation, and policy experts from Rush University Medical Center, University of Chicago Medicine, the Illinois Health and

Hospital Association, and the Commonwealth Fund. Mount Sinai is among the 147 hospitals and health centers around the country that submitted surveys in the first cohort. The Racial Health Equity Report, a free web-based survey assessing 34 metrics to be completed annually following a baseline assessment, measures performance in addressing racial health disparities and organizational-level inequities. The report is intended to promote collective improvement within healthcare organizations while allowing for the development of national best practice standards for achieving health equity. The report scores and ranks key metrics related to people, the organization, patients, and the community, with progress measured from "not in place" (no plans yet discussed) to "best practice" (the practice has been implemented and is tracked, and the process and associated data are considered a best practice).

The Racial Health Equity Progress Report offers a standardized approach, and the results serve as institutional and national benchmarks, says Doran Ricks, MSN, RN, MBA, and Vice President for Data Quality and Stewardship for the Mount Sinai Health System. "With the help of the Road Map Strategy Leads across the health system, we were able to map our strategies onto the survey metrics. We found the process of completing the survey, as well as the results, useful as a way both to measure our progress in achieving Road Map goals, as well as to consider other metrics of importance to us at Mount Sinai." This national initiative provides an excellent tool and helpful resources for healthcare organizations to guide the aggregation, organization, and interpretation of health equity efforts.[3,7]

---

## Recommended Reading and Resources

Association of American Medical Colleges. Anti-racism Resources. Accessed February 2, 2025. https://www.aamc.org/about-us/equity-diversity-inclusion/anti-racism-resources://

Blackstock U. *Legacy: A Black Physician Reckons with Racism in Medicine.* New York: Viking; 2023.

Blue Cross and Blue Shield of Massachusetts Foundation. Health Equity Action Toolkit. December 2023. https://www.bluecrossmafoundation.org/sites/g/files/csphws2101/files/2023-12/Health_Equity_Toolkit_Dec23_FINAL.pdf

Illinois Health and Hospital Association. Racial Equity in Healthcare: Progress Report Playbook: From Data to Action. October 2022. https://www.compdatainfo.com/getmedia/efa132d7-fadb-48e6-bcd1-beb0e8c8f18e/IHA-Racial-Equity-playbook-10-14-22.pdf. Accessed December 31, 2024

Institute for Diversity, Health, and Equity. The Health Equity Roadmap. American Hospital Association. Chicago, Illinois. Accessed March 29, 2025. https://equity.aha.org/

Nelson CR, Marsh DS, Noor S, Liu N. Racial health equity plans, a how-to manual. Local and Regional Alliance on Race & Equity. Haas Institute for a Fair and Inclusive Society. University of California, Berkeley. 2016. https://www.racialequityalliance.org/viewdocument/racial-equity-action-plans-a-how-t

Rise to Health Coalition. Health Care Organizations. Actions & Activities Resources. https://risetohealthequity.org/sites/default/files/2024-12/Rise%20to%20Health%20Coalition%20Action%20and%20Activities%20Resources_FINAL.pdf

Rush University Medical Center. Racial Health Equity Progress Report. Accessed February 2, 2025. https://www.rush.edu/about-us/rush-community/rush-bmo-institute-health-equity/racial-health-equity-progress-report

Winters M-F and the Winters Group. *Racial Justice at Work. Practical Solutions for Systemic Change*. Berrett–Koehler; 2023.

## References

1. Purdie-Greenaway V, Davidson MN. Is D&I about us? How inclusion practices undermine Black advancement and how to design for real inclusion. In: Morgan Roberts L, Mayo AJ, Thomas DA, eds. *Race, Work, and Leadership: New Perspectives on the Black Experience*. Harvard Business Review Press; 2019: 312–322.
2. Bryant AS, Healey JA, Wilkie S, Carten C, Sequist TD, Taveras EM. A health system framework for addressing structural racism: Mass General Brigham's United Against Racism Initiative. *Health Equity*. 2023 Sep 13; 7(1):533–542. https://doi.org/10.1089/heq.2023.00771
3. Butts GP, Abner P, Hess L, Palermo AS, Cotilletta B, Gianelle A, et al. Designing a Road Map for Action to Address Bias and Racism within a large academic medical center. *Acad Med*. 2023; 98(12):1381–1389. https://doi.org/10.1097/acm.00000000000052892
4. Lapiner C, Heron N, Rustgi AK, Armstrong KA, Lantigua RA, Williams OA, et al. Institutional approach to anti-racism in health and health care. *BMJ Leader*. 2023 Nov 15; 7:1–5. https://doi.org/10.1136/leader-2023-0008223
5. Wilkins CH, Williams M, Karapreet K, DeBraun MR. Academic medicine's journey toward racial equity must be grounded in history: Recommendations for becoming an antiracist academic medical center. *Acad Med*. 2021 Nov: 96(11). https://doi.org/10.1097/acm.00000000000043744

6. Curren R, Nelson J, Marsh DS, Noor S, Liu N. Racial equity action plans, a how-to manual. Haas Institute for a Fair and Inclusive Society, University of California, Berkeley. 2016. https://www.racialequityalliance.org/resources/racial-equity-toolkit-opportunity-operationalize-equity/5
7. Illinois Health and Hospital Association. Guidance Document for the Racial Equity in Healthcare Progress Report. June 2021. https://www.team-iha.org/quality-and-safety/health-disparities-resource-hub/6
8. Kania J, Kania M. Collective impact. *Stanf Soc Innov Rev.* 2011; 9:36–41.
9. Kania J, Junious W, Paul S, Sherri B, Mark K, Splansky JJ. Center equity in collective impact. *Stanf Soc Innov Rev.* 2022; 20:38–45.
10. Kaner S. *Facilitator's Guide to Participatory Decision-Making.* 3rd ed. San Francisco: Jossey–Bass; 2014.
11. Ansell DA, Oliver-Hightower JD, Goodman LJ, Lateef OB, Johnson TJ. Health equity as a system strategy: The Rush University Medical Center framework. *NEJM Catalyst.* 2021; 2(5). https://doi.org/full/10.1056/CAT.20.06747
12. Seattle Children's. Health Equity and Anti-racism Action Plan. September 2021. https://www.seattlechildrens.org/about/commitment-anti-racism8
13. Coalition of Communities of Color. Tool for Organizational Self-Assessment Related to Racial Equity. 2014. Portland, Oregon. https://www.coalitioncommunitiescolor.org/research-and-publications/cccorgassessment
14. Vanderbilt University Medical Center. Racial Equity Plan. Updated May 2022. https://www.vumc.org/healthequityinclusiveexcellence/sites/default/files/public_files/VUMC%20Racial_Equity_Plan%20For%20Release.pdf
15. American Institutes for Research. Aligning Systems with Communities to Advance Equity Through Shared Measurement. Guiding Principles. 2021. https://www.air.org/project/cross-sector-measurement-advance-health-equity9
16. Muhamed KG, Cardo Rodriguez A. Antiracist institutional change in healthcare: Antiracism and Accountability (IARA) project. Harvard Kennedy School. 2023. https://ash.harvard.edu/resources/antiracist-institutional-change-in-healthcare/
17. Blackstock U. *Legacy: A Black Physician Reckons with Racism in Medicine.* New York: Viking; 2023.
18. Wang ML, Gomes A, Rosa M, Copeland P, Santana VJ. A systematic review of diversity, equity, and inclusion and antiracism studies: Findings and future directions. *Transl Behav Med.* 2024; 14:156–171. https://doi.org/10.1093/tbm/ibad061

# 2

# Embedding Equity into Quality Measurement

The laudable but elusive goal of eliminating *health disparities*, defined as preventable differences in the burden of disease, injury, violence, or opportunities to achieve optimal health that are experienced by socially disadvantaged populations, is a complex societal undertaking that will require redress of historical and contemporary injustices in education, employment, housing, transportation systems, and access to capital, as well as attention to commercial and political determinants of health. These go far beyond the province of any single sector. However, the elimination of *healthcare disparities* is completely within the purview of healthcare professionals and organizations.

Healthcare disparities may be defined as "racial or ethnic differences in the quality of healthcare that are not due to access-related factors or clinical needs, preferences, and appropriateness of the intervention or treatment."[1] The Agency for Healthcare Research and Quality has tracked core measures of quality and access annually since 2002. The 2023 National Healthcare Quality and Disparities Report reveals that racial and ethnic disparities in quality persist. For the most recent data year, American Indian or Alaska Native people had worse quality of care than White people for 44% of quality measures; Asian people received worse care than White people for 35% of quality measures; Black people received worse care than White people for 52% of quality measures; Native Hawaiian/Pacific Islander people received worse care than White people for 36% of quality measures; and Hispanic people received worse care than non-Hispanic White people for 37% of quality measures.[2]

Addressing disparities in health and health care is important not only from an equity standpoint, but also for improving the nation's

*Transforming Health Care*. Lynne D. Richardson and Sima Rabinowitz, Oxford University Press.
© Oxford University Press (2026). DOI: 10.1093/oso/9780197805374.003.0003

overall health and economic prosperity. People of color and other underserved groups experience higher rates of illness and death across a wide range of health conditions, limiting the overall health of the nation.[3] Research further finds that health disparities are financially costly, resulting in excess medical care costs and lost productivity, as well as additional economic losses due to premature deaths each year.[4]

Healthcare organizations have both moral and legal responsibilities to deliver equitable care to all of the patients they serve. Fulfilling these responsibilities requires that healthcare organizations transform themselves into institutions that value everyone equally and that provide the same quality of care to everyone, regardless of the race, ethnicity, language preference, gender, religion, socioeconomic status, or ability of the patient. Healthcare organizations must commit to achieving equitable outcomes across all groups, with focused and ongoing efforts to eliminate practices and policies that are rooted in racism throughout their organizations, and to prevent bias and discrimination in every encounter.

The next three chapters detail many of the processes and policies involved in delivering high-quality, equitable clinical care. We begin with a discussion of how to use existing strategies and resources while transforming quality improvement processes into a robust method of identifying and monitoring disparities in care.

## Using Quality Data to Measure the Equitableness of Clinical Care

Every healthcare organization in the United States spends substantial time and effort measuring the quality of the care it delivers. Quality metrics assessing clinical processes and patient outcomes are collected, recorded, analyzed, and reported for every aspect of care. The massive amounts of data generated by these activities are used by clinical and administrative staff throughout the organization to monitor safety and effectiveness, continuously improve quality and performance, and fulfill regulatory and contractual reporting requirements. These same data can be used to determine whether the organization is providing the same quality of care to all patients. Healthcare leaders should not assume that this is already happening in their organizations; they must ensure that it does by incorporating the measurement of equity into quality measurement throughout the enterprise.

## Collecting Accurate and Complete Data on Patient Race, Ethnicity, and Language Preference

For more than a decade, healthcare organizations have been required to collect patient-level data on race, ethnicity, and language preference (REL),[5] but despite the regulatory mandates, many healthcare organizations do not have complete and accurate REL data for all of their patients.[6,7] Patients should be asked for their REL data by front-desk staff, and only self-reported data should be entered into the hospital's information systems. Managers and staff may be reluctant to ask patients for this information, fearing that patients will be offended. The rationale for collecting REL data should be explained to staff and shared with patients. With proper training and scripting, staff can learn to successfully collect these data with very low refusal rates.[8] If a patient responds with "*Why are you asking me that?*" the staff member explains: "*We collect this information so we can make sure that we are providing the same quality of care to all of our patients.*"

A benchmark of acquiring accurate, self-reported data on more than 95% of patients can be achieved by any healthcare organization through an organization-wide performance improvement program that begins with structured training of all registration staff, both inpatient and outpatient. Guessing about a patient's race, ethnicity or language preference (observer assignment) based on their appearance or their name is unacceptable. If a patient is unable to answer for themselves, then a relative or caregiver may be asked: "*How does this patient usually describe themselves?*" At the outset, staff should be trained to ask everyone, including patients for whom REL data are already in the organization's information system, so that they may correct inaccurate data that were previously entered before self-report became standard procedure.

Ongoing performance improvement tools should be used to monitor progress toward the goal of 95% completeness for each practice, unit, or facility, with supervisors being held accountable for attaining and maintaining the goal. Missing data or responses such as "unknown," "not asked," or "not available" are counted as incomplete. Resources, both in-person trainings and online training modules, should be developed to train new employees and to retrain/remediate individual front-desk staff members who fall below the 95% benchmark.

Many electronic health records (EHRs) allow for greater granularity than the federal categories for race (American Indian or Alaska Native, Asian, Black or African American, Middle Eastern or North African, Native Hawaiian/Pacific Islander, White) and ethnicity (Hispanic, non-Hispanic). It is important to include a racial category of "Other" because many Latine individuals will not self-report a race and instead identify themselves only by their ethnicity. Allowing the collection of more detailed REL data from all of the patient populations served by the organization will inform efforts to provide culturally competent, patient-centered care. For example, rather than simply recording a patient's ethnicity as Hispanic, allow them to identify themselves as Puerto Rican, Cuban American, Dominican, Mexican American, etc. Similarly, rather than just recording a patient's race as Asian, capture information about whether their background is Chinese, Japanese, Korean, Vietnamese, Cambodian, Indian, Pakistani, etc. These smaller subgroups can be electronically distributed into the federal categories needed for regulatory reporting.

Some institutions are now collecting self-reported REL data, as well as data on sexual orientation and gender identity (SOGI) and other social determinants, through the patient portal of their EHR. This may enhance data collection among some groups, but should not be a substitute for appropriately training front-desk staff to collect this information from all patients.

## Examining Existing Quality Metrics for Each Racial, Ethnic, and Linguistic Group

Collecting accurate and complete REL data from all patients is the essential first step to monitoring equity as part of quality. Once this is accomplished, an organization can use the quality data that are already being generated to examine and compare the quality of care provided to different groups simply by stratifying the quality data by patient race, ethnicity, and language preference. This will allow the systematic identification of disparities in care across various demographic groups. This may be an uncomfortable process since most clinicians and healthcare professionals believe that they provide equitable care. Often, complacency, or the idea that "everyone is treated the same," is a reflection of the mistaken belief that the norms and values of the dominant culture are universally applicable. Providing equitable care requires not only recognizing differences between cultures but also valuing those differences and customizing care to meet each patient's needs. Examining the quality data for each REL group served will provide empirical evidence, rather than mere opinion, regarding the presence of disparate care in a particular setting. Once it is determined that some subpopulations are more likely to receive poorer-quality care, specific quality improvement interventions can be developed to address the identified disparities.[9]

Quality metrics include both process measures (vaccination rates, preventive screenings, recommended follow-up visits) and outcome measures (mortality, hospitalization, readmission rates). Differences in process measures for REL groups represent healthcare disparities that must be addressed by the healthcare organization. If, for example, Black women in a particular primary care practice are not receiving recommended breast cancer screening with mammograms at the same rate as White women in the practice, the healthcare organization must address this disparity in care. More information will be required to select the appropriate intervention. If they are not being referred for the screening, a provider-focused intervention may be needed. If they are being referred but not getting the screening, barriers to obtaining a mammogram need to be identified and eliminated: Is the service only offered on weekdays from 9:00 a.m. to 5:00 p.m., requiring some women to miss work to obtain the procedure? Are interpreter services not available at the imaging facility to accommodate patients with limited English proficiency? Is the screening being explained in a way that makes it likely that some women will not accept the referral? Multiple quality improvement initiatives or interventions may be required to address each of these issues.

Many institutions now use dashboards that are built on patient-level databases to track performance and trends in their quality metrics. Linking patient-level REL data to the clinical data allows easy visualization of differences in quality metrics and facilitates tracking changes over time as quality improvement initiatives to address identified disparities are rolled out.

Unlike differences in process measures, differences in outcome measures for REL groups may not be due, or not solely due, to disparities in the quality of care provided. Patient outcomes are affected by many factors other than the health care delivered. For example, inpatient mortality is influenced by the patient's age, their comorbid conditions, the severity of illness at the time they presented for care, etc., in addition to the health care provided by the hospital. Determining whether a difference in mortality between REL groups reflects a disparity in care requires risk-adjusted analyses that include all factors known to influence mortality before characterizing the difference as a disparity in care that needs to be addressed by the healthcare organization. However, if unwarranted variations in diagnostic or treatment choices by providers are influencing patient mortality, those disparities in care must be addressed.

## Implementing Quality Improvement Initiatives to Address Disparities in Care

Many of the tools routinely used to improve performance and enhance quality can be tailored and targeted to address REL disparities in care. Tools to influence provider behavior such as EHR-embedded clinical decision support, audit feedback, and performance incentives could be used to address the previous example of disparities in breast cancer screening. Implementing evidence-based clinical guidelines and pathways often has the double benefit of improving quality for all patients while decreasing disparities in care by minimizing clinician variation that may be fueled by implicit or explicit biases. Patient-facing interventions such as patient navigators and care coordination programs can be used to provide support and overcome barriers to obtaining care for patients who are experiencing disparities in care. It is especially important to identify system-level barriers to providing equitable care and dismantle them so that all patients receive high-quality care throughout the organization.

Once targeted interventions have been implemented to address identified disparities, their effectiveness can be monitored by tracking quality metrics for the groups receiving disparate care. Baseline performance and progress toward REL equity can be tracked for each facility or practice, and even for individual providers. Giving individual and practice-wide feedback is a pillar of quality improvement practices; these strategies can be effectively applied to the elimination of care disparities. Identifying best-performing providers and provider groups may help in identifying best practices that can be disseminated using quality improvement techniques.

## The Social Determinants of Health

Identifying the social determinants of health (SDOH) for both individuals and communities has been an issue of increasing importance for healthcare organizations of all types since they were first defined nearly a quarter of a century ago as "the conditions in which people are born, grow, work, live, and age."[10] (See Table 2.1) It is important to clarify that the social, commercial, political, and environmental determinants or drivers of health can be positive (conferring benefit or advantage) or detrimental (conferring harm or disadvantage). Many adverse SDOH (unstable housing, food insecurity, low levels of educational attainment, exposure to violence, etc.) are downstream effects of deeply rooted upstream forces, principally structural racism, which create both individual- and neighborhood-level health risks and individual health-related social needs (HRSN). The role and responsibility of healthcare organizations in assessing and responding to patients' HRSN, and the best practices for doing so, are complex issues driven by the evolving national healthcare regulatory landscape, competing interests and priorities, significant logistical constraints, and local contexts, among other factors.

It is important to understand the concept of "needs" in this context as basic material and social necessities (food and shelter, safety and

**Table 2.1** Social Determinants of Health.

| **Personal Characteristics** | **Economic Stability and Financial Resources** | **Education** |
|---|---|---|
| Race | Employment | Highest grade completed |
| Ethnicity | Income | High school diploma |
| Age | Debt/Wealth | College |
| Sex/Gender | Food security/ insecurity | Graduate school/ professional school |
| Sexual orientation/ Gender identity | Housing insecurity/ instability | Vocational training |
| Preferred language | Homelessness | Literacy |
| Disability status | Utilities (heat, water, electricity) | Digital literacy |
| Veteran status | Childcare access and affordability | Health Literacy |
| Refugee/immigration status | | |
| Incarceration status | | |
| **Neighborhood and Physical Environment** | **Community and Social Context** | **Health Care** |
| Availability of healthy food | Racism | Insurance coverage |
| Availability of clean water | Bias and discrimination | Availability of/access to primary care |
| Housing quality | Sexism | Availability of/access to specialty care |
| Access to parks, playgrounds | Social support | Health literacy |
| Interpersonal safety/violence | Social isolation | Language interpretation services |
| Neighborhood safety/violence | Stress | |
| | Xenophobia | |
| | Homophobia | |
| | Social capital | |
| | Collective efficacy | |

*continued*

**Table 2.1** *continued*

| **Neighborhood and Physical Environment** |
| --- |
| Public transportation |
| Exposure to outdoor pollutants |
| Exposure to indoor toxins |
| Broadband access |

*Note*: Adapted from multiple sources on SODH and social needs screening tools:
Center for Health Equity Advancement. Health Disparities and Social Determinants of Health. University of Pennsylvania. Philadelphia, PA. https://www.chea.upenn.edu/health-disparities-and-social-determinants-of-health/
Healthy People 2030, U.S. Department of Health and Human Services, Office of Disease Prevention and Health Promotion. Social Determinants of Health. https://odphp.health.gov/healthypeople/objectives-and-data/social-determinants-health
National Association of Community Health Centers, Inc., Association of Asian Pacific Community Health Organizations, and Oregon Primary Care Association. 2016. The PRAPRE® Screening Tool. https://prapare.org/the-prapare-screening-tool/
Social Interventions Research and Evaluations Network (siren). Social Needs Screening Tool Comparison Table. University of California, San Francisco. 2019. September 2024. https://sirenetwork.ucsf.edu/tools-resources/resources/screening-tools-comparison

social connection, etc.) that may be lacking or inadequate. A discussion of need necessarily centers around what is missing. Nonetheless, we want to emphasize that HRSN should not be framed as deficits, either for individuals or for communities. An antiracist approach to transforming care demands that we identify and respond to HRSN in the context of inequitable access to, and distribution of, fundamental material and social resources. At the same time, in alignment with the imperative to rectify prior harms as a fundamental component of antiracist practice and achieving racial health equity, it would be unethical, at the very least, to ask patients about their needs yet do nothing to help address them in some way. For this reason, any program of HRSN screening must include plans and mechanisms for responding on some level to the specific needs identified. We will see in Chapter 3 that these strategies can vary significantly by setting, population, resources, regulations, and, above all, the needs to be addressed.

## Screening for HRSN

The development and implementation of HRSN screening programs engages health and hospital systems in overlapping issues and concerns with implications for equity. Most clinicians understand that social needs are directly related to health but may lack the ability (expertise, time, resources) to address these needs. Until recently, few healthcare organizations screened for all key "social drivers of health structural measures" as initially defined by the Centers for Medicare & Medicaid Services (CMS)[11] and piloted through its Accountable Health Communities model.[12] Some hospitals and physicians' practices do not screen for any.

### Screening Tools

Screening for the social drivers of health is a priority in CMS's newly implemented Framework for Health Equity, with assessment and reporting required for every inpatient during every stay and the total rate of positive screens for all patients for: (1) food insecurity, (2) housing instability, (3) transportation needs, (4) utility needs, and (5) interpersonal safety.[13] In addition to estimating the impact of HRSN on healthcare utilization and evaluating the quality of care, one of the goals of screening is to identify individuals who will benefit from engagement with community-based service providers, and for this reason, hospitals are required to provide referrals to community resources.

Given the enormous variability in hospitals and their patient populations, as well as differing levels of expertise and experience with screening implementation, CMS allows health and hospital systems to select screening tools (although evidence-based tools are encouraged) and methods, including the specific questions to be asked for each social need, and the mechanisms for referring patients to resources. The screening tool created for the Accountable Health Communities (ACH) model initiative (19 screening items across 13 domains) is recommended, although not required.[14] The CMS screening tool is available in 11 languages; however, at least one other validated tool, PRAPARE®, is available in at least 25 languages and could be more suitable depending on an organization's patient population.[15] Hospitals may also use ICD-10 Social Determinants of Health Z codes to capture social driver information if they have used these codes to screen for HRSN in ambulatory settings and if they capture the required information. For health and hospital systems, standardizing and coordinating inpatient and ambulatory HRSN screening processes, data collection, and mechanisms for referrals to social care programs and services require attention to issues of equity in their design, implementation, and evaluation.

On the one hand, flexibility in the choice of screening tools may allow for the development of highly tailored, patient-engaged, and hyperlocal screening and referral programs, which may be more effective in addressing patients' individual needs. On the other hand, vague guidance and a lack of national standards could further deepen disparities. Questions that are too broadly articulated or that reflect cultural insensitivity, for example, may obscure rather than elucidate patients' real day-to-day needs and could result in links to inappropriate or inadequate services or damage trust. Data that are not harmonized across sites or organizations could result in imprecise or inaccurate views of social needs nationally and/or locally, resulting in the inefficient or ineffective allocation of resources. Further, CMS does not require reporting of race, ethnicity, or other demographic data as a part of SDOH screening, but healthcare organizations will clearly need to integrate these types of data.

In 2023, the Joint Commission incorporated six measures of health equity into its overall safety accreditation standards.[16] Distinct from CMS, the Joint Commission allows hospitals to determine which HRSN to include in screening and, notably, includes difficulty paying for care (prescriptions and medical bills) among the short list of representative core needs. The Joint Commission also offers a rigorous Health Equity Certification program, with certification available for inpatient and acute hospitals, ambulatory sites, and behavioral health centers. The Commission's Health Equity Certification Resource Center provides guides, fact sheets, links to validated screening tools, toolkits, and case studies, as well as materials related to other aspects of the equitable delivery of care, which may be useful for any healthcare organization that is implementing or expanding HRSN screening programs, even for those that are not seeking certification.[17]

The focus on screening for social determinants or drivers has intensified given the changing regulatory landscape and evolving payor models. Nonetheless, screening for social needs is not new to many healthcare organizations, and tools and strategies have been adapted and implemented in a range of settings (primary care, emergency departments, pediatric clinics, family medicine practices, and inpatient units). Extensive resources exist on social needs screening produced or aggregated by a variety of organizations; these include guidance on integration of HRSN data in EHRs; adapting social needs screening tools for local contexts; operations and workflow; training and education for clinicians, nurses, allied health professionals (social workers, community health workers), and staff; and development of referral resources. We have included several useful resources in the Recommended Reading and Resources list at the end of this chapter.

## Implementing HRSN Screening

Each of these areas (choice of tool; decisions around who will administer screening, where, when, and how; etc.) involves complex issues in the context of equity. As with the collection of REL data, staff must understand the purpose of screening and receive appropriate training. There is a danger that HRSN screening programs may reinforce or exacerbate discriminatory attitudes and behaviors when they are not grounded in equitable principles and frameworks or if they are implemented without appropriate education and training. Patients should be informed that they can elect not to participate in screening or decline to answer specific questions. Clear communication, appropriate language (several screening tools are available in multiple languages), and literacy levels are important factors. Screening questions may need to be adapted for local contexts and populations. Cultural humility and sensitivity are fundamental in administering screening (as they are for all interactions). Digital access and literacy must be considered where screening may be integrated into online patient portals. Healthcare organizations will want to both convene coordinated teams (administrators, clinicians, staff) that are equipped with the right resources and engage patient stakeholders every step of the way in designing and evaluating screening if these programs are to meaningfully identify patients' social care needs.

Providing patient-centered care requires that healthcare organizations acquire a deep understanding of their patients' characteristics, cultures, and HRSN. Once organizations have implemented a robust system of collecting accurate patient REL data and have incorporated the use of REL data into their quality improvement program, data on patients' HRSN can provide insight into the mechanisms underlying certain care disparities and may inform potential interventions to deliver more effective care and achieve more equitable outcomes.

## Summary

1. Collect accurate patient-reported REL data. Staff should understand the rationale and be trained to share the rationale with patients, if asked. The completeness of REL data should be monitored for each unit or practice within the organization, with retraining and remediation if REL data are not available for at least 95% of patients.
2. Stratify existing quality metrics by race, ethnicity, and preferred language. REL data should be added to all quality dashboards, and quality committees and councils should routinely examine the quality of care provided to Black, Latine, and Native patients, as well as to other socially disadvantaged groups.
3. Identify disparities in the quality of care being delivered. Differences in process measures (vaccination rates, preventive screenings, recommended follow-up visits) for REL groups represent healthcare disparities that must be addressed by the healthcare organization. Differences in outcome measures (mortality,

hospitalization, rehospitalization) for REL groups require risk-adjusted analyses that also include all other factors known to influence the outcome (age, comorbidities) before characterizing the difference as a healthcare disparity that needs to be addressed by the healthcare organization.

4. Implement evidence-based solutions to address any disparities identified. Patient-focused, provider-focused, and systems-level interventions should be considered. Conduct systematic evaluation of interventions using rigorous performance improvement techniques.
5. Screen for HRSN. Carefully consider the choice of screening tool, staff procedures, and training, and use information on HRSN to inform strategies to eliminate care disparities.

**SPOTLIGHT**

## An Institutional Quality Scorecard to Measure Healthcare Equity

*The Quality Scorecard is part of an enterprise-wide plan to create and model a culture of equity in which we collaborate to identify and reflect on the ways our organization may contribute to health inequities and works to eliminate them.*

James Williams Jr., MA; Vice President, Diversity, Equity, and Inclusion; Urban Health Initiative, University of Chicago Medical Center

At the University of Chicago Medical Center (UCMC), equity and quality are inextricably linked. As part of an interconnected, organization-wide set of strategies to build a culture of equity, a data science and analytics team; diversity, equity, and inclusion leaders; and the UCMC's quality committee collaborated to create an interactive institutional quality scorecard to track and measure healthcare equity with a focus on improving the health of groups that have been historically marginalized. The intensive process began with an assessment of clinical priorities and development of a suite of dashboards, followed by in-depth review and analysis by UCMC's quality committee, whose members include physician quality chiefs from every clinical department and service line, directors from the chief medical officers' teams, select house staff, a board member, administrative and clinical leaders, and members of the diversity, equity, and inclusion department. The scorecard stratifies more than 100 key performance metrics by various patient demographics (age, gender, race, ethnicity, zip code, preferred language, sexual orientation, gender identity, and payor) and operational dimensions, which adds depth to the equity analysis and the questions that can be asked. Measures include inpatient and ambulatory care outcomes, as well as patient experience data, and the dashboards allow users to view trends over time and performance relative to institutional targets.

Following an initial targeted rollout, the scorecard is now available to all UCMC healthcare clinicians, staff, and faculty. The data science and analytics team provides training to help users understand both the scorecard's functionality (how it works) and the data (how results can be interpreted to identify inequities). Given the amount and complexity of the data, coupled with enormous interest in leveraging the scorecard to problem solve and drive action, determining the ways in which people across the organization are using the data is an ongoing process. "Democratizing the data is about more than making the data available and accessible," says Mary Kate Selling, MHA, Chief Analytics Officer. "We need to be sure that people know how to look at the data to uncover what's going on clinically."

The quality scorecard continues to evolve. New demographic data are being integrated (sexual orientation and gender identity, for example), and additional quality measures will be incorporated. "It takes a large, coordinated effort and sufficient time to do this work well. Equity is an issue of quality, and for quality, you need accurate data and users who know how to make use of it," says Mark Connolly, Director of the Business Intelligence Program.

Patients are also key partners in UCMC's equity work and play an integral role in quality improvement efforts. Initiatives are underway to transform models of care that employ patient-informed approaches in priority areas such as chronic disease management. Another important aspect of the project has been integration of demographic filters in the Social Needs Screening dashboard to help address social determinants of health. Together, scorecard data and the voice of patients will drive quality, equity, and innovation.

> *When we consider multiple variables together—sociodemographic data with clinical data by unit or service, for example—a bigger picture emerges. Then we can ask how these factors intersect to create relevant differences that, working together with our patients, we can begin to address.*
>
> Scott Cook, PhD, Founding Co-Director, the Robert Wood Johnson Foundation Advancing Health Equity: Leading Care, Payment, and Systems Transformation Program, University of Chicago Medical Center

---

## Recommended Reading and Resources


American Association of Family Physicians. The EveryONE Project Toolkit. April 2024. https://www.aafp.org/family-physician/patient-care/the-everyone-project/toolkit.html

Connolly M, Selling MK, Cook S, Williams JS Jr., Chin MH, Unscheid CA. Development, implementation, and use of an equity lens integrated into an institutional scorecard. *JAMIA.* 2021; 28(8):2785–1790. https://doi.org/10.1093/jamia/ocab082

Migita D, Cooper A, Barry D, Bettinger B, Tieder A, Sharek PJ. Equity dashboards: Data visualizations for assessing inequities in a hospital setting. *Pediatrics.* 2023 Mar 1; 151(3):e2022058848. https://doi.org/10.1542/peds.2022–058848

National Association of Community Health Centers. PRAPARE® (Protocol for Assessing and Responding to Patients Assets, Risks, and Experiences). Bethesda, Maryland. https://prapare.org/

Pillai D, Artiga S. Revisions to federal standards for collecting and reporting data on race and ethnicity: What they are and why do they matter? Kaiser Family Foundation. April 30, 2024. https://www.kff.org/racial-equity-and-health-policy/issue-brief/revisions-to-federal-standards-for-collecting-and-reporting-data-on-race-and-ethnicity-what-are-they-and-why-do-they-matter/

University of California, San Francisco. Social Interventions Research and Evaluations Network (SIREN). Evidence and Resource Library. https://sirenetwork.ucsf.edu/tools/evidence-library

## References


1. Institute of Medicine (US) Committee on Understanding and Eliminating Racial and Ethnic Disparities in Health Care; Smedley BD, Stith AY, Nelson AR, eds. *Unequal Treatment: Confronting Racial and Ethnic Disparities in Health Care.* National Academies Press; 2003. https://doi.org/10.17226/12875
2. Agency for Healthcare Research and Quality. 2023 National Healthcare: National Healthcare Quality and Disparities Report: Report Appendices. December 2023; AHRQ Pub No. 23(4)-0091-EF. https://www.ahrq.gov/research/findings/nhqrdr/nhqdr23/index.html
3. Ndugga N, Hill L, Artiga S. Key data on health and healthcare by race and ethnicity. Kaiser Family Foundation. June 11, 2024. https://www.kff.org/key-data-on-health-and-health-care-by-race-and-ethnicity/?entry=executive-summary-introduction
4. Altarum. The Business Case for Racial Equity: A Strategy for Growth. April 24, 2018. https://altarum.org/news-and-insights/business-case-racial-equity-strategy-growth
5. American Recovery and Reinvestment Act of February 17, 2009. Pub L. No. 111-5. 123 STAT 115. https://www.congress.gov/111/plaws/publ5/PLAW-111publ5.pdf
6. Douglas MD, Dawes DE, Holden KB, Mack D. Missed policy opportunities to advance health equity by recording demographic data in electronic health records. *Am J Public Health.* 2015 Jul; 105 (Suppl 3):S380–S388. https://doi.org/10.2105/AJPH.2014.302384
7. James CV, Haley JM, Allen EH, Nelson T. *Using Race and Ethnic Data to Advance Health Equity.* Urban Institute. October 2023. https://www.urban.org/sites/default/files/2023-10/Using%20Race%20and%20Ethnicity%20Data%20to%20Advance%20Health%20Equity.pdf
8. Vega Perez R, Hayden L, Bickell N, Abner P, Richardson LD, Ngai Ka Ming. Improving patient race and ethnicity data capture to address health disparities: A case study from large urban health system. *Cureus.* 2022 Jan 5;14(1):e20973. https://doi.org/10.7759/cureus.20973
9. Health Research and Educational Trust. Improving health equity through data collection and use: A guide for hospitals. American Hospital Association. March 2011. https://www.aha.org/system/files/2018-02/improving-health-equity-data-collection-hospital-leaders-2011.pdf
10. World Health Organization. Social Determinants of Health. Accessed February 8, 2025. https://www.who.int/health-topics/social-determinants-of-health#tab=tab_1
11. Centers for Medicare & Medicaid Services. CMS Quality Reporting and Value-Based Programs & Initiatives. Updated August 2024. https://mmshub.cms.gov/about-quality/quality-at-CMS/quality/programs
12. Centers for Medicare & Medicaid Services. Accountable Health Communities Model. Accessed February 8, 2025. https://www.cms.gov/priorities/innovation/innovation-models/ahcm
13. Centers for Medicare & Medicaid Services. Hospital Quality Reporting Program. Frequently Asked Questions: Social Drivers of Health Measures. April 2024. https://www.qualityreportingcenter.com/globalassets/2024/04/iqr/17.-sdoh-measure--faqs_april-2024_vfinal508.pdf

14. Centers for Medicare and Medicaid Innovation. The Accountable Health Communities Health-Related Social Needs Screening. Centers for Medicare & Medicaid Services. Accessed February 8, 2025. https://www.cms.gov/priorities/innovation/files/worksheets/ahcm-screeningtool.pdf
15. National Association of Community Health Centers. PRAPARE® (Protocol for Assessing and Responding to Patients Assets, Risks, and Experiences). Bethesda, Maryland. https://prapare.org/
16. The Joint Commission. Health Care Equity. Accessed February 2, 2025. https://www.jointcommission.org/our-priorities/health-care-equity/
17. The Joint Commission. Health Care Equity Certification Resource Center. Provision of Care. https://www.jointcommission.org/our-priorities/health-care-equity/certification-resource-center/provision-of-care/#t=_StrategiesTab

# 3

# Embedding Equity into Care Delivery

There is growing recognition among clinicians and healthcare leaders that disparities in the delivery of care are not merely common, but also widespread and that these disparities are driven largely by structural racism and the social determinants of health (SDOH).[1] As we saw in Chapter 2, health and hospital systems are developing equity-focused methods to identify population-level disparities in care quality that may be linked to clinical activities and patient outcomes. Assessing the practices, processes, and policies that result in inequitable treatment is a critical first step. However, this information is only meaningful if we use it to transform the way care is delivered. We must apply an antiracist, equity lens to every aspect of care delivery in every setting, from communicating with and about patients, to providing access to their electronic health records through patient portals, to assessing and responding to their health-related social needs (HRSN).

## Addressing the Social Drivers of Health and Health Equity

In Chapter 2, we discussed the regulatory responsibilities healthcare organizations have to screen for HRSN. However, screening is just the first step; patients with HRSN must have those needs addressed. For healthcare organizations that lack the infrastructure to provide direct services, collection of SDOH from patients should trigger appropriate referrals to community-based organizations that can provide the services or resources required to address the identified needs or risks. Healthcare organizations must also learn to use information on social

*Transforming Health Care*. Lynne D. Richardson and Sima Rabinowitz, Oxford University Press.
 DOI: 10.1093/oso/9780197805374.003.0004

determinants to inform clinical care and treatment decisions for individual patients and, at the macro level, to redesign care delivery systems to accommodate the social, economic, and physical conditions in which their patients are born, grow, work, live, and age.

It is important to understand that social determinants operate at both individual and community levels to affect a wide range of health outcomes and risks. Personal factors such as race, income, and education interact with neighborhood factors such as poor housing stock, environmental toxins, violence, and food access to impact health. Screening for HRSN is a prerequisite to providing access to social care resources that may help improve individual patients' lives, although screening and referral will not change the structural factors responsible for the conditions that gave rise to these needs in the first place. The shift in the expansion of value-based payments that incentivize prevention and improved health has created growing pressure on healthcare providers and organizations to address health-related factors that are outside the healthcare system. It is difficult to envision achieving health equity without working to address these underlying structural issues while attending to the individual social needs that impact health and well-being.

## Assessing Population Risk versus Individual Needs

A focus on health equity and value-based payment models, among other factors, has driven interest in the use of SDOH data to inform population health strategies. A growing number of companies market and sell business analytics programs designed to provide actionable insights into the impact of specific social drivers on health outcomes and their associated costs or risks. These analytics are based on data aggregated from a variety of public and private sources that leverage proprietary systems and technologies for the purpose of helping healthcare organizations predict population-level risk for specific health conditions (e.g., chronic illness) and healthcare utilization (e.g., hospital readmissions or visits to the emergency department). These analyses may link specific social determinants with key healthcare delivery challenges, identifying targets for enhanced care coordination or discharge planning, based on the prevalence of a particular risk in a given geographic area. There is significant variation in the size of the geographic areas for which such data are available (county, zip code, census tract).

It is important to distinguish between leveraging aggregated SDOH data and population-level health strategies to improve outcomes and reduce costs for the long term and assessing a patient's individual HRSN at the point of care. When using community-level data to stratify risk or predict which groups will require specific types of support or services, we may miss or misunderstand individual patients' needs and, in so doing, uphold or exacerbate stereotyping and discriminatory practices, which can lead to unintended (and undesirable) consequences. Community-level data can be used to target population-level interventions or can be incorporated into risk adjustment models to account for baseline differences in health status; regardless of the granularity of the community-level data (county, zip code, census tract, census block), it is important to remember that these data should not be used to impute characteristics about any individual who is residing in that geographic area.

Many healthcare organizations also develop their own prediction models to identify patients who are at increased risk for social needs. These models often involve integrating patient-level data from electronic health records with community-level data. As risk prediction models, these strategies—combining individual patient and community-level data or indices to create social risk scores—may be less prone to assign risk where none exists or to miss needs that should be addressed. Here, again, it is important to avoid assumptions about an individual patient's needs or to draw conclusions based on data that were intended primarily to inform population-level assessments and strategic decision-making.

## Building Bidirectional Referral Systems

Both the Centers for Medicare & Medicaid Services (CMS) and the Joint Commission require that patients be screened for HRSN and that those who screen positive be offered referral resources to local community organizations that provide direct services or serve as referral hubs. As we have emphasized, screening patients for HRSN must be understood as one component of an integrated strategy, which includes links to resources (internal or external) that are appropriately matched to identified needs. Despite the growing recognition that safe housing, healthy food, access to transportation, and other basic needs can dramatically affect one's health, there is no organized system for addressing these needs. There is, rather, a patchwork of programs, providers, initiatives, and funding streams that vary significantly from place to place. Many communities face large gaps and shortages in social services and community programs (long intake waiting lists, frequent staff turnover, resource constraints), which can make accessing and receiving services difficult.

The standard of care in many healthcare organizations has been to provide patients with a printed list of community-based resources, often without additional support or follow-up. Patients' overlapping social needs may compromise their ability to access services. Individuals who screen positive for transportation to medical appointments may also lack transportation to access a food pantry or to meet with intake workers at a social services agency. Intersecting needs should, ideally, be addressed together. Screening and referral programs without mechanisms for postreferral follow-up lack information not only about the impact or outcomes of a referral on an individual patient's health, but also about which services and programs are effective overall.

Health and hospital systems around the country have developed strategies to optimize the referral process by connecting patients with social workers or community health workers to help further clarify patients' specific needs and support access to services, sometimes through automated referral platforms that aggregate local resources. As we will describe in later chapters on equity-focused business practices, workforce and human resources strategies, and public health and policy initiatives, the most impactful approaches are likely to involve collaborative, multisector engagement and partnerships.

An emerging but promising collaborative approach is the development of closed-loop systems: digital platforms with automated referral mechanisms that can match and link patient records across sectors, allowing for bidirectional communication between healthcare organizations and a network or hub of community-based partners. Community-based organizations (CBOs) track intake, utilization, and resolution or persistence of needs; these data are then integrated into the patients' electronic health records to create a unified view of screening, linkage to resources, and results.

Standing up a bidirectional referral network is a resource-intensive endeavor. Developing productive partnerships takes time; managing data privacy issues, the customization of electronic health records, and interoperability issues require specialized expertise. Many community-based organizations lack the technical infrastructure to participate without assistance to build capacity and require financial resources (and, potentially, case-by-case reimbursement) to manage the demands that a bidirectional process places on both staff and information systems. Nonetheless, with the establishment of strong networks and proper funding, closed-loop systems may represent the best opportunity to help improve health through social care integration.

Whatever the choice of screening and referral tools and strategies to address HRSN, applying an equity lens requires centering patients' lived experience, tailoring processes and programs to accommodate the patients being served, working to minimize the potential for unintended adverse consequences, and promoting understanding of the imperative to address social needs to rectify historical and current inequities in the distribution of, and access to, fundamental opportunities and resources.

## Developing and Delivering Social Care Programs and Services

Increasingly, healthcare organizations and hospital systems are engaging and investing in a range of strategies to address patients' social needs directly through the provision of programs and services (on-site food pantries and produce markets, shuttle services and hospitality vans), investment in partnerships with local community organizations and businesses (vouchers for local farms or community gardens, ride-sharing programs, transit passes), and co-location of services (legal–medical and financial–medical partnerships). In addition to the obvious and substantial challenges associated with limited or complete lack of coverage and reimbursement for social care interventions, as well as critical issues associated with data privacy and security, healthcare organizations and hospital systems that provide or partner to provide social care activities also face a complex regulatory environment. Federal and state policies and regulations may govern which social care activities can be included in healthcare services or how free and discounted services may be promoted, depending on how they are financed.[2,3]

Social care interventions vary substantially in size and scope, from the distribution of vouchers for food or utilities to the development of transitional housing facilities, and clearly must be designed around highly specific local or regional needs and resources. In Chapter 7, we will consider multisector initiatives to address economic well-being at the community level. We will focus briefly here on several innovative, co-located services, which bring or develop expertise on-site in healthcare organizations to help address individuals' and families' nonmedical needs: specifically, medical–legal partnerships (MLPs), medical–financial partnerships (MFPs), and hospital-based violence prevention interventions.

## Embedding Medical–Legal Partnerships

Co-location of legal or financial services is an emerging trend in health and social care integration. Medical–legal partnerships (MLPs) have been embedded in more than 450 healthcare organizations in nearly every state in both urban and rural settings, including in children's hospitals, federally qualified health centers, Veterans Administration medical centers, safety-net hospitals, and academic medical centers.[4] Healthcare organizations partner with Legal Aid, law schools, and private law firms to provide pro bono services ranging from a single consultation to full legal representation to address health-harming legal needs related to housing (evictions, housing repairs); access to public benefits; employment; family law; education rights; immigration (protection of legal status); affirming the rights of lesbian, gay, bisexual, transgender, nonbinary, queer, or questioning individuals; and advance planning (power of attorney, guardianships), among others. Legal partners also provide training for clinicians and staff (how to screen for legal needs, for example) and educational workshops for individuals and families.

MLPs provide services to patients and families who would often otherwise lack access to an attorney and who may have multiple legal needs that impact their health or, inversely, whose health may impact their ability to manage their legal situation. They have shown measurable health benefits, such as improvements in diabetes management and mental health, as well as benefits for healthcare organizations, including reductions in spending on high-needs patients, hospitalizations, and emergency department visits.[4,5] Beyond the economic benefit for healthcare organizations, financial outcomes for individuals and families could include healthcare debt elimination or other tangible benefits, such as restoration of utilities or increased access to Supplemental Security Income.

## Embedding Medical–Financial Partnerships

Medical–financial partnerships (MFPs) integrate clinical and financial services to address financial strain and improve financial well-being as a health promotion activity. MFPs have been embedded in pediatric primary care and family health clinics in response to the high rates of poverty in children in the United States and the resulting impact on health over the life course. Programs and services may include free on-site assistance with tax preparation (the earned income tax credit, for example) and benefits programs (Supplemental Nutrition Assistance/SNAP Program), financial literacy training, credit score counseling, emergency finance solutions, and financial coaching. Assessment of financial stress in one form or another (food insecurity, difficulty paying for utilities, employment status, medical debt, etc.) is a component of all validated HRSN screening tools, and screening questions can be adapted for the population, including language and setting.

Healthcare organizations can work with the Internal Revenue Service to register as a volunteer income tax assistance (VITA) provider. Health and hospital systems that offer economic services often collaborate with community-based organizations and nonprofit agencies to staff their on-site programs. In conjunction with, or in place of, on-site services, some MFPs employ the type of closed-loop referrals model described earlier in this chapter, with targeted links to off-site services or virtual programs and feedback from partners about utilization and outcomes. Similar to Medicaid programs, tax, finance, and public benefits programs and regulations vary by state, making it essential to partner with local experts.

MFPs have been successful in helping generate substantial payments from earned income tax credits, a federal program for families that have low to moderate income that is considered an important poverty alleviation tool, and in helping individuals and families increase savings, reduce debt, and increase enrollment in public benefits and banking programs (e.g., the Low-Income Home Energy Assistance Program, 529 college savings accounts).[6] A goal of MFPs is to build trust with families to promote sustained engagement with healthcare providers, and MFPs are associated with improved clinic attendance and vaccination rates.[6] Patients are especially interested in these types of programs, which provide support both for managing complex administrative processes and tangible benefits. Like many of the initiatives described throughout this book, MFPs represent a novel model of care developed through cross-sector collaborations and coalitions and designed for impact beyond the clinical setting.

## Addressing an Urgent Public Health Issue: Hospital-Based Violence Intervention Programs

Gun violence is a leading cause of premature death among adults and the number one cause of death among children and adolescents in the United States, with disproportionate impact on people of color.[7] In 2024, U.S. Surgeon General Vivek Murthy declared firearm violence a public health crisis,[8] although this declaration was removed from government websites early in 2025.

Like all forms of violence (including intimate partner violence and child abuse), gun violence has an enormous impact on health beyond physical injury, not only for the survivors of violence but also for their families and the larger community. Firearm injuries account for billions of dollars in initial medical costs (emergency department visits, inpatient hospitalizations) every year.[9] Moreover, an individual who has been injured by intentional interpersonal violence is twice as likely to be violently injured again than someone who has never experienced such violence.[10]

Hospital-based violence intervention programs (HVIP) integrate the expertise of violence-prevention specialists—typically through community-based organizations—and healthcare providers. HVIPs support the health and broader social needs of survivors and their families with the goal of reducing the risk of reinjury and improving physical and mental well-being. Interventions include screening in the emergency department, at the patient's bedside, or in ambulatory care settings, as appropriate, followed by long-term case management and wraparound services, including crisis intervention. The HVIP approach is a way of reframing violence as a preventable healthcare concern that can be addressed by partnering with communities, including survivors of violence, and that can yield impact beyond individual needs. At least 85 cities in the United States have HVIPs; these programs are shown to reduce the risk of reinjury and hospitalization and their associated costs.[11] Unfortunately, funding remains a significant barrier because Medicaid only covers these programs in a handful of states, and future changes to Medicaid may erode funds for existing efforts.

From an equity perspective, providing programs and services to mitigate threat and harm (unmet legal needs, financial stress, physical violence) demonstrates an understanding of safety and security as integral to health and, therefore, to the delivery of quality health care. Such programs and services can serve to empower people who have been, and continue to be, marginalized and disenfranchised and to unify concepts of personal and societal health and well-being.

## Healthcare Redesign to Accommodate the Impact of Social Adversity

In addition to providing resources to address identified social needs, social determinants data should be used by healthcare organizations to inform individualized treatment plans and care models that accommodate the circumstances of the patient. This will require operational changes and innovations that disrupt the current provider-centric system, such as extended hours, co-location of medical and social services, telehealth, and remote patient monitoring, all delivered by service-oriented, culturally competent clinicians and staff. At the macro level, healthcare delivery processes and workflows must be redesigned to address patients' requirements and preferences. Healthcare organizations must shift the focus from helping people fit into the current care delivery system to one where the care delivery system is redesigned to serve people where they live, work, learn, play, or receive health care. The current approach to health care requires considerable effort and skill to obtain needed services; those who are not well positioned and equipped to navigate the delivery system are often systematically left out.

The U.S. healthcare system is exorbitantly expensive but yields the poorest health outcomes compared to other developed countries. Transforming health care to improve the access, quality, and affordability of care for everyone will require a consumer-centric focus that leverages innovative use of digital and technology enablers to provide evidence-based care and thoughtful care coordination. Systems science must guide the completion of the shift to value-based care with a focus on prevention, health promotion, and outcomes-based care models. This redesign will require the engagement of not only clinical and administrative leaders, but also patients, caregivers, employers, payors, and policy makers to build a new healthcare ecosystem that is both equitable and sustainable.[12]

## Communicating Equitably: Language and Literacy

An issue of enormous importance for the equitable delivery of care is communication. Nearly half of all healthcare workers and more than 70% of Latine healthcare workers say they have witnessed discrimination against patients who predominantly speak a language other than English.[13] At the same time, health literacy in the United States is exceptionally poor overall, and many adults, regardless of their level of education, have limited health literacy skills—the skills needed to obtain and understand basic information about health and healthcare services to make health-related decisions. A high degree of organizational health literacy—communicating spoken, written, or electronically conveyed health information in a way that is clear, free of medical jargon, and usable in English or in a patient's preferred language—is critical to deliver high-quality care to everyone.

## Limited English Proficiency and Language Preference

Every state in the United States has thousands to millions of speakers of non-English languages, with nearly 70 million individuals (approximately 20% of the U.S. population) who speak a language other than English at home and approximately 27 million individuals (about 8% of the U.S. population) who communicate in English "less than very well."[14] Individuals who speak English less than very well are classified in the U.S. Census as having limited English proficiency. They have been protected by law from discrimination on the basis of preferred language or ability to speak English and are entitled to language services to ensure effective communication with healthcare providers and insurers.[15]

Although these laws were first enacted in 1964, a recent final rule, in place at the time of the writing of this book, extends to the provision of care in virtually every healthcare organization in the U.S. healthcare system and includes both on-site and telehealth services.[16] The same laws also protect individuals with hearing and/or sight impairment who may require various forms of language assistance services (American Sign Language interpretation, tactile interpretation, print materials in Braille), which are all, in fact, covered under the same ICD billing code (although reimbursement, as we will describe shortly, is extremely limited). We should note that the term limited English proficiency is problematic on many levels, not the least of which is lack of clarity about the concept of proficiency, and where possible, it may be preferable, from an equity perspective, to use terms that emphasize language preference rather than proficiency.

### Language Assistance Services

Providing access to appropriate language interpreter services is critical to improve care for these patients. Individuals who are classified as having limited English proficiency have higher rates of mortality, longer hospital stays, increased rates of adverse inpatient experiences (such as falls and postsurgical infections), higher rates of revisits to emergency departments, and lower medication adherence, and they very often have a poor patient experience.[17] There is, however, a tremendous gap between need and access, at least in part because of payor models. Commercial insurers are not required to reimburse for language interpretation services, and Medicare does not cover these services. As of the writing of this book, Medicaid and the Children's Health Improvement Program (CHIP) reimburse for language interpretation services in only 17 states and the District of Columbia, typically with strict limits on visit length; even in states that offer coverage, language interpreter services are underutilized.[16]

Only a relatively small percentage of patients with limited English proficiency receive professional language interpretation services, which may be delivered in person, over the phone, via video remote interpreting, or through "automated" translation (speech or text-based machine translations). Even fewer have access to a language-concordant physician (where the patient and physician share a preferred language or have in common a language in which both are proficient). The law does not stipulate how language interpretation services must be provided, but does require that interpreters be "qualified," meaning that they must be proficient in English and at least one other target language, able to interpret or translate specialized terms, and committed to client confidentiality. Many healthcare organizations rely on "ad hoc" interpreters, a patient's family or friends, or a staff member who possesses some level of proficiency in English and in the patient's preferred language. This approach has the potential to significantly detract from the quality of care delivered while potentially compromising privacy and confidentiality. Ad hoc interpreters may lack familiarity with medical terminology or have little or no experience navigating the healthcare system.

To ensure that patients whose preferred language is not English receive the highest-quality care, and as described in Chapter 2, healthcare organizations should capture "preferred" (sometimes classified as "primary") language, along with other demographic data, and this information should be accessible to providers throughout the organization. Next, it is important to consider the various settings and points along the care trajectory where interpreters may be needed—in the clinic, at the bedside, in an imaging suite or rehabilitation facility—as well as valid translations of consent forms, discharge papers, and instructions related to care. Healthcare organizations should let patients know about their language assistance services, plan for these services in advance when possible, and track utilization. Staff training around nondiscrimination policies and language assistance procedures is required by law, but healthcare organizations may want to consider additional training for clinicians and staff on how to work with interpreters effectively and how to communicate respectfully with patients who do not speak English proficiently or whose preferred language is not English.

Professional language assistance services (whether provided in-house or contracted through third-party vendors), although expensive in the short term, can have long-term benefits for both patients (increased patient satisfaction and improved outcomes) and healthcare organizations. Providing appropriate language services can reduce costs by decreasing readmission rates, among other economic benefits.[18] Redesigning care to meet the needs of patients whose preferred language is not English presents an opportunity to engage this patient population in the design of language access initiatives, which could, for example, include having patient focus groups test the comprehensibility of translated patient education materials or the effectiveness of telephone versus video interpretation in the context of different settings.

Advancing equity in language access is difficult to imagine without changes to payor models and policies. Healthcare leaders who are committed to equity in care should consider advocating for legislation to fund qualified, professional language assistance services; prioritizing resources for such services within their organizations; and measuring progress in the provision of these services as a part of achieving equity goals.

## Health Literacy

Health literacy is not solely an issue of individual skill level and knowledge. Healthcare organizations must provide health information in a way that is easy for patients to find, comprehend, and use to make health-related decisions. Yet, health information is often communicated in a way that is complex, confusing, or easily misinterpreted, and medical and health system jargon is difficult for many people to understand, regardless of their educational background.

Limited health literacy can result in miscommunication that contributes to longer hospital stays, increased emergency department use, medication errors, poor management of chronic conditions, and the associated costs for health and hospital systems.[19] Similar to providing high-quality care to patients with a non-English-language preference, advancing equity in health literacy requires an understanding of how communication impacts care in different settings and across the care continuum, from online appointment booking to hospital signage and from prescription labels to urgent public health messages.

Many healthcare organizations have adopted "health literacy universal precautions," a model of care in which all patients are assumed to be at risk of not understanding information that is of relevance to their health. "Universal" in this context does not mean identical or uniform. In fact, recognizing that every patient is at risk of not understanding makes clearer the importance of tailoring communication to address patients' distinct needs. Because personal health literacy skills are largely determined by education, a social driver of health with significant disparities in access and quality, employing health literacy universal precautions may, in fact, be an effective strategy for advancing equity. Universal precautions are grounded in health-literate approaches such as employing plain language, presenting numerical data in more easily understood formats, encouraging questions, using the teach-back method, and providing staff with training to communicate clearly, among other strategies, which should also include language access and culturally sensitive approaches.

Assessing health literacy requires cultural sensitivity, consent if formal literacy assessments will be conducted, and language-appropriate tools (for patients whose preferred language is not English). Training and resources for clinicians and staff to improve health literacy and patient-centered communication strategies should include practical guidance and examples. Developing written materials for patients is another area where patient engagement can be effective; patient input can help healthcare providers create materials that are more accessible, relevant, and readable. Above all, healthcare leaders must understand that addressing basic health literacy is a fundamental component of care and should be a priority for healthcare organizations that are committed to achieving equity.

## Optimizing Electronic Health Record Patient Portals for Equity

The core concerns around communicating equitably—health literacy, language access, bias-free and culturally sensitive provider/patient interactions and patient education—extend to online tools and apps such as electronic health record patient portals, where they merge with questions of inclusive access and digital literacy. *Are all patients offered access to the portal? Do all patients understand how to use it? Does the portal support a multilingual interface? Have patients and caregivers been engaged in helping to design, test, and evaluate this tool?* Healthcare organizations that are committed to achieving the equitable delivery of care may want to establish a digital equity council or committee, including patient advocates and community leaders, to consider these types of questions and help ensure that digital initiatives prioritize fairness and accessibility.

We know that disparities in use decrease when patients are offered access to portals and encouraged to use them. Ensuring that healthcare providers raise awareness of the tool and promote use among all patients can contribute to equity in portal participation. Many patients prefer, or only have access to, mobile apps, making it essential for patient portals to be designed for mobile use; and many patients may need assistance to download an app and learn how it works. Educating patients about the benefits of using a portal and addressing concerns about privacy, security, and confidentiality are key to sustained engagement.

Although hospitals and clinics often rely on their staff to provide this support to patients, another option is to engage digital health navigators, an emerging model for improving digital health literacy that can be deployed across multiple settings. Trained digital health navigators, often community health workers (CHWs), promote use of the portal and deliver personalized education to increase participation and improve the patient experience. Healthcare organizations with closely integrated digital functions can help boost engagement by automating a post-discharge or post-visit message or text with an activation code for the portal.

Patient portals can contribute to equity efforts by connecting patients with culturally and linguistically appropriate education materials tailored to address patients' specific health conditions and well-being needs and goals. These might include videos, podcasts, and links to relevant websites, as well as written materials. Finally, patient portals may potentially be used to connect patients with community resources, using the kinds of closed-loop approaches described in Chapter 2. Personalizing these resources can help build trust and encourage engagement. Patient portals, like many digital health tools, have the potential to improve the quality of care and patient experience, if not health outcomes. However, they may just as easily exacerbate inequities if they are not designed to reduce barriers to access and use and to reduce patient burden.

## Engaging Patients in Improving Care

Partnering with patients and their families and caregivers to improve the quality of care is essential to achieving equity. Patient experience—assessing individual patients' perceptions of and views on the care they have received—although critical, is separate from engagement, which involves patients and their families/caregivers in creating change. Healthcare organizations often engage patients and families/caregivers as members of formal Patient and Family Advisory Councils (PFACs) or other types of patient advisory councils, and less commonly as members of organizational committees (quality councils, for example) or workgroups. Patient engagement in quality improvement ranges from collaboration on smaller-scale projects, such as redesigning signage or revising a set of patient educational materials, to systems transformation. As we recommended in Chapter 1, healthcare organizations should consider including patients in antiracism road map or action plan task forces and committees.

## Strategies to Promote Equity in Patient Engagement

Applying an equity lens to patient engagement requires, first and foremost, a commitment to centering patients' voices and appreciating their role as experts on their own experience. There is clearly a great deal to be learned from patients, both individually and collectively, and it is important to raise awareness throughout the organization about the value of patient engagement, as well as to create accountability. Administrators, clinicians, and staff all need to gain an understanding of why patient engagement matters and how it will be operationalized.

### Inclusion of Patients and Families

Equity-focused patient engagement requires the representation and inclusion of individuals and groups who have been marginalized and excluded, especially those who will be most impacted by the specific initiatives being undertaken, along with options and opportunities for meaningful participation. These include both the types of activities in which patients are engaged and making appropriate accommodations to facilitate participation, such as stipends or other forms of compensation, reimbursement for transportation or transit passes, meals, provision of child care, and convenient scheduling of meetings and activities.

To support representation and inclusion on patient and family/caregiver councils, boards, committees, and workgroups, healthcare organizations should provide language services, as needed, during meetings and events and for all relevant communications. It may be helpful to create virtual or hybrid (on-site and online options) opportunities, particularly where scheduling or transportation would otherwise make participation difficult. Meaningful patient engagement is an investment in safety and quality and, as such, requires the resources (budget, staffing, administrative support) to be effective.

## Meaningful Participation, Engagement Principles, and Governance

Equity-focused, authentic patient engagement involves more than soliciting opinions or feedback on changes once they have been implemented or on projects nearing completion. Patient and family/caregiver partners can participate in identifying issues, challenges, and priorities and in co-designing solutions and evaluating them. Patient and family/caregiver groups have, for example, helped to develop an intervention to reduce wait times in a primary care clinic,[20] design a program to avoid hospital readmissions by improving care transitions from hospital to home for patients who have had a hip fracture,[21] implement strategies for the dissemination of information about COVID-19 testing sites,[22] and create and cofacilitate training for a hospital's customer service teams to improve interactions with patients.[23]

Although patient and family/caregiver councils and committees vary significantly from organization to organization and even within health and hospital systems (larger systems may have multiple patient advisory groups, with membership by population or health condition), a few equity-focused principles are broadly applicable. Patient engagement is more impactful when it is linked with organizational equity and inclusion initiatives and with organizational goals and priorities and when it is embedded into the structure of the organization rather than siloed; a patient quality council could, for example, be included in organizational charts.

Ongoing patient and family boards or councils should be chaired or co-led by a patient or family/caregiver member, and patient and family/caregiver members should help lead or co-lead discussions or presentations. When patients are included as members of standing organizational committees, such as hospital safety and quality boards or performance improvement committees, it is important to avoid token representation and to consider ways to fully integrate patient and family/caregiver members and facilitate their involvement. Recruitment for patient engagement should be ongoing so that new voices continue to be included. Orientation activities, training, and ongoing learning opportunities for patients and family/caregivers can help support active involvement and retention and may also be useful for clinicians and staff who have not previously collaborated in patient engagement.

## Evaluating and Sustaining Engagement

It is imperative to conduct formal evaluations of patient engagement, include patients and family/caregivers in the process, and share the results. Members of patient and family/caregiver engagement groups and initiatives want to know how their work has contributed to improvements in the delivery of care, impacted the organization, or motivated advocacy and policy initiatives. Trust, respect, and transparency (sharing information, reporting results, acknowledging both successes and where efforts fall short) are essential to advance equity.

Leaders and managers can demonstrate an organization's commitment to patient engagement by ensuring that staff have the time and resources needed to devote to work related to patient engagement, receiving regular updates on patient engagement efforts, and meeting with patients and family/caregivers to learn about their experiences, perspectives, and priorities. Highlighting patient-informed innovations and changes to programs, processes, practices, policies, services, and facilities—and, where feasible, any associated outcomes—sends the message that partnering with patients is a pathway to improvement and high-quality care.

Patient engagement can also be a way of deepening partnerships with communities. Healthcare organizations may want to engage community leaders in recruiting patients and families/caregivers to participate in patient engagement initiatives. Members of patient and family/caregiver boards and councils may, in turn, partner with community organizations and groups on outreach and education efforts or lead or participate in community-focused health campaigns or events. Robust patient engagement efforts may help build and sustain relationships with communities that can extend beyond care delivery, for example, to the types of workforce initiatives described in Chapter 5 or the community development collaborations described in Chapter 7.

## Summary

1. In each clinical setting, conduct HRSN screening in a systematic way that avoids stereotyping. Poorly implemented methods of capturing social determinants data may simply codify bias within health systems and have a negative impact on vulnerable populations.
2. Avoid making assumptions or guessing about patients' individual HRSN based on neighborhood-level data that are intended to inform population-level assessments and decision-making.
3. When leveraging information technology, ensure that digital approaches to integrating social care into health care do not increase existing health disparities as a result of the "digital divide" between affluent and under-resourced populations.
4. When screening for HRSN, employ a mechanism for referring patients to appropriate resources to address identified needs. Collaborative approaches created in partnership with community-based organizations may be most effective.
5. Use information on social determinants to inform clinical care and treatment decisions for individual patients and, at the macro level, to redesign care delivery systems to accommodate the social adversity that constrains patients' abilities to use healthcare services.
6. Provide language interpreter services to patients whose preferred language is not English and strive to consider language preference, as well as health literacy, in every aspect of treatment, including in the design of patient portals.
7. Engage patients in quality improvement efforts through participation on patient and family advisory committees and organizational committees or workgroups. Equity-focused engagement requires the representation and inclusion of individuals and

groups who have been marginalized and who will be most impacted by specific improvement initiatives.

## SPOTLIGHT

### Helping Families Improve Financial Well-Being

*An enormous number of people across the country experience financial strain, which is central to health. We need to provide economic services as a routine part of care, not as something we just research, and not only at safety net hospitals, but everywhere.*

Lucy E. Marcil, MD, MPH; Cofounder and Executive Director, StreetCred; Associate Director of Economic Mobility, Center for the Urban Child and Healthy Family, Boston Medical Center; Associate Professor of Pediatrics, Boston University Chobanian & Avedisian School of Medicine

Financial strain, or the economic challenges that result from financial instability, debt, or poor credit, can take a huge toll on health. Evidence-based approaches to intervene exist but are significantly underutilized, says Dr. Lucy Marcil. At Boston Medical Center, the largest essential hospital in the region, Dr. Marcil and her colleagues have developed an economic services bundle that is offered to patients as a routine part of pediatric primary care. Since its launch in 2016 with a single service, earned income tax credit tax preparation assistance, StreetCred has led to more than 6,000 families claiming more than $14 million in tax refunds. The on-site program now offers a set of seven services, including tax preparation assistance; enrollment in the Supplemental Nutrition Assistance Program and the Special Supplemental Nutrition Program for Women, Infants, and Children and access to the medical center's on-site food pantry; and engagement in asset-building tools, such as 529 college savings accounts, paid family and medical leave, and a federal Family Self-Sufficiency Program. The services are introduced to families at a newborn visit by a financial navigator who follows up with brief check-in calls to build trust and sustain contact and again during clinic well-baby visits in the first year of life. An update to the program is in progress, including the possibility of offering services during prenatal visits, with the goal of improving maternal and child health earlier in pregnancy. Every patient in the clinic is offered these services, if a financial navigator is available, and StreetCred maintains a strict no-screening policy, an approach that is intended to eliminate stigma and encourage participation.

Many organizations in the financial sector are open to building medical–financial partnerships, but Dr. Marcil emphasizes that it is essential to work with partners to do more than simply connect patients to public services. The provision of co-located tax assistance programs (at the clinic) is not especially costly or complex to establish. Navigator-based models that offer intensive coaching and networking to individuals or groups on bundled services can be more costly, but the financial and health benefits for families are incalculable. The StreetCred team has developed a group coaching model with an unexpected impact—participants found social networking with peers to be among the most meaningful aspects of the experience, and some groups have opted to continue even after formal coaching sessions have ended.

StreetCred has established an open-source collaborative—the Health by Wealth Collective—that offers free logistical support and guidance to healthcare organizations across the country that are working to integrate economic services into the delivery of care and advance their economic justice model. Dr. Marcil says, "Financial stress is the norm, and we often don't know what adversity people are facing. Reducing financial stress as a health promotion strategy is an evidence-based approach to care for our patients."[24]

---

## Recommended Reading and Resources

American Hospital Association Physician Alliance. Patient and Family Advisory Councils blueprint. A start-up and strategy guide. American Hospital Association. January 2022. https://www.aha.org/system/files/media/file/2022/01/alliance-pfac-blueprint-2022.pdf

Center for Health Care Strategies. Health Literacy Fact Sheets. March 2024. https://www.chcs.org/resource/health-literacy-fact-sheets/

Health Begins. RO1 and Community Health Investment. RO1 Calculator. Accessed February 3, 2025. https://healthbegins.org/expertise/#health-social-care-integration

The Joint Commission. Quick Tip #13: Overcoming Challenges to Providing Quality Care to Limited English Proficient Patients. October 2021. https://www.jointcommission.org/resources/news-and-multimedia/newsletters/newsletters/quick-safety/quick-safety--issue-13-overcoming-the-challenges-of-providing-care-to-lep-patients/overcoming-the-challenges-of-providing-care-to-lep-patients/

National Center for Medical–Legal Partnership. The Milken Institute School of Public Health. George Washington University. Accessed February 2, 2025. https://medical-legalpartnership.org/partnerships/

Nicholas LM, Waidman TA, Clemans-Cope L, Garrett B, Taylor K. Tracing value from social determinants solutions. *Health Aff Sch.* 2025; qxae173. https://doi.org/10.1093/haschl/qxae173

University of California, San Francisco. Social Interventions Research and Evaluations Network (SIREN). Evidence and Resource Library. Accessed February 25, 2025. https://sirenetwork.ucsf.edu/tools/evidence-library

## References


1. Bees J. How health care leaders view disparities in care. *NEJM Catalyst Innov Care Deliv.* 2024; 5(6). https://doi.org/10.1056/CAT.24.0211
2. National Academies of Sciences, Engineering, and Medicine. *Integrating Social Care into the Delivery of Health Care: Moving Upstream to Improve the Nation's Health.* National Academies Press; 2019. https://doi.org/10.17226/25467
3. Sandu S, Landauer R, Katz MC, Gottlieb L. Underestimated challenges for social care initiatives. *N Engl J Med.* 2024; 390(19):1737–1739. https://doi.org/10.1097/MLR.0000000000006433
4. National Center for Medical–Legal Partnership. The Milken Institute School of Public Health. George Washington University. Accessed February 2, 2025. https://medical-legalpartnership.org/partnerships/
5. Johnson DY, Asay S, Keegan G, Wu L, Zietowski ML, Zakrison TL, et al. US medical–legal partnerships to address health-harming legal needs: Closing the health justice gap. *J Gen Intern Med.* 2024 May; 39(7):12–4–121. https://pubmed.ncbi.nlm.nih.gov/38191972/#:~:text=Abstract,needs%20with%20civil%20legal%20remedies
6. Gusoff G, Schickedanz A. Addressing economic drivers of health in the clinic: The role and potential of medical–financial partnerships. *J Appl Res.* 2023; 14(2):Article 2. https://digitalcommons.library.tmc.edu/childrenatrisk/vol14/iss2/2/#:~:text=Gusoff%2C%20Geoffrey%20and,10.58464/2155%2D5834.1524
7. Center for Gun Violence Solutions. Gun violence in the United States. Examining the burden among children and teens. Johns Hopkins Bloomberg School of Public Health. September 2024. https://publichealth.jhu.edu/sites/default/files/2024-09/2022-cgvs-gun-violence-in-the-united-states.pdf

8. U.S. Department of Health and Human Services. Firearm Violence in America. Accessed February 2, 2025. https://www.hhs.gov/surgeongeneral/reports-and-publications/firearm-violence/index.html
9. The National Institute for Healthcare Management. Gun Violence: The Impact on Society. July 2, 2024. https://nihcm.org/publications/gun-violence-the-impact-on-society
10. Jang A, Thomas A, Slocum J, Tesorero K, Danna G, Saklecha A, Wafford E, Regan S, Stey AM. The gap between hospital-based violence intervention services and client needs: A systematic review. *Surgery*. 2023; 174:1008–1020. https://doi.org/10.1016/j.surg.2023.07.011
11. The Health Alliance for Violence Intervention. The HAVI Position Brief. Hospital-Based Violence Intervention: Practices & Policies to End the Cycle of Violence. September 2023. https://www.thehavi.org/healthcare-advocacy
12. Erwin K, Krishnan JA. Using design methods to provide the care that people want and need. *J Comp Eff Res*. 2016; 5:13–15. https://doi.org/10.2217/cer.15.624pmid:266988285
13. The Commonwealth Fund African American Research Collaborative. Revealing Disparities: Health Care Workers' Observations of Discrimination Against Patients. February 15, 2024. https://www.commonwealthfund.org/publications/issue-briefs/2024/feb/revealing-disparities-health-care-workers-observations6
14. U.S. Census Bureau. American Community Survey: Selected Social Characteristics in the United States 2022. https://data.census.gov/table/ACSDP1Y2022.DP02?q=DP027
15. U.S. Department of Health and Human Services. Limited English Proficiency. Accessed February 19, 2025. https://www.hhs.gov/civil-rights/for-individuals/special-topics/limited-english-proficiency/index.html
16. Youdelman M. What is required under Title VI and Section 1557 to ensure language access for individuals with limited English proficiency? National Health Law Program. May 9, 2024. https://healthlaw.org/resource/what-is-required-under-title-vi-and-section-1557-to-ensure-language-access-for-individuals-with-limited-english-proficiency/8
17. Twersky SE, Jefferson R, Garcia-Ortiz L, Williams E, Pina C. The impact of limited English proficiency on healthcare access and outcomes in the U.S.: A scoping review. *Healthcare*. 2024 Jan 31; 12(3):364. https://doi.org/10.3390/healthcare12030364
18. Karliner LS, Pérez-Estable E, Gregorick SE. Convenient access to professional interpreters in the hospital decreases readmission practices and hospital expenditures for patients with limited English proficiency. *Med Care*. 2017; 55(3):199–206. https://doi.org/10.1097/MLR.0000000000006439
19. Coughlin SS, Vernon M, Hatzigeorgiou C, George V. Health literacy, social determinants of health, and disease prevention and control. *J Environ Health Sci*. 2020; 6(1):3061. Epub 2020 Dec 16. PMID: 33604453; PMCID: PMC7889072
20. Sharma AE, Willard-Grace R, Willis A, Zieve O, Dubé K, Parker C, et al. "How can we talk about patient-centered care without patients at the table?"—Lessons learned from patient advisory councils. *JABFM*. 2016; 29(6):775–784. https://doi.org/10.3122/jabfm.2016.06.150380
21. Baker GR, Fancott C, Judd M, O'Connor P. Expanding patient engagement in quality improvement and health system redesign: Three Canadian case

studies. *HealthC Manage Forum.* 2016; 29(5):176–182. https://doi.org/10.1177/0840470416645601

22. Woodward EN, Melgar Castillo AI, True G, Willging C, Kirchner JE. Challenges and promising solutions to engaging patients in healthcare implementation in the United States: An environmental scan. *BMC Health Serv Res.* 2024; 24:29. https://doi.org/10.1186%2Fs12913-023-10315-y
23. Institute for Patient- and-Family-Centered Care. Profiles of Change. Children's Specialized Hospital. Accessed February 19, 2025. https://www.ipfcc.org/profiles/childrens-specialized.html
24. Boston Medical Center. StreetCred. Accessed February 19, 2025. https://www.bmc.org/streetcred

# 4

# Eliminating Bias and Racism from Care Delivery

It is important to recognize that structural racism is not simply the accumulation of individually held prejudices; rather, it is the embodiment of racism in rules, laws, practices, policies, and organizational approaches. Structural racism manifests in healthcare organizations and health systems in multiple disturbing ways. Care for racial/ethnic minorities is generally reimbursed at lower rates and often provided in settings that are chronically underresourced. Diagnostic algorithms and devices may result in systematic harm to certain groups. The organization of ambulatory practices and the use of digital health technologies may serve to create or exacerbate inequities in treatment and outcomes. To dismantle structural racism in a healthcare organization requires a thorough understanding of these phenomena, a deep commitment to becoming an antiracist organization, and careful evaluation of interventions to alter structures, processes, and outcomes that are inequitable. The first step is to identify and quantify the myriad ways that bias and racism are embedded throughout the healthcare delivery system, several of which we will describe in this chapter.

## Practice Segregation

Although legal segregation was abolished decades ago, de facto segregation persists in many aspects of society, including healthcare institutions and systems. Many hospitals did not admit Black patients or allow Black physicians to join the medical staff until well into the 20th century. This led to separate medical systems for non-White populations until the 1964 Civil Rights Act made the racial segregation of

*Transforming Health Care*. Lynne D. Richardson and Sima Rabinowitz, Oxford University Press.
© Oxford University Press (2026). DOI: 10.1093/oso/9780197805374.003.0005

healthcare institutions illegal. Nevertheless, racial/ethnic segregation currently exists in multiple forms within healthcare settings. Nominally, such segregation is based on insurance, but socioeconomic status is very strongly related to race/ethnicity as a result of decades of diminished educational, occupational, and economic opportunities for certain racial and ethnic groups. Disparate access to health insurance among Blacks and ethnic minorities results in certain healthcare organizations having disproportionate numbers of uninsured and Medicaid patients; this causes chronic underresourcing because Medicaid reimbursement is significantly lower than that of commercial insurance. Teaching services in academic medical centers are often located in areas that have a disproportionate number of socially and economically disadvantaged residents, codifying the care of these individuals by less experienced providers.

Segregation in ambulatory healthcare settings takes several forms, including physically separate sites with different staffing and resources for different groups of patients, as well as internally segregated "teaching" practices where attending physicians may see commercially insured patients while students, residents, and fellows see Medicaid and uninsured patients. Healthcare organizations may see this as providing access to disadvantaged populations without acknowledging the parallels to the failed "separate but equal" doctrine that characterized the U.S. education system for most of the 20th century. Perverse incentives and discriminatory insurance programs help to perpetuate the maintenance of separate outpatient practices for indigent patients.

There are both direct and indirect health impacts of segregation in health care. Direct effects include unequal access to certain medical services and providers and systematic differences in the quality of care provided, leading to disparate health outcomes, including mortality. Indirect impacts of segregated practices include perceived discrimination and mistrust of healthcare providers and systems by those who are relegated to practices that serve socially and economically disadvantaged populations. Healthcare organizations that are committed to becoming equitable, antiracist organizations must find financially viable ways to unify practices and services rather than continuing to provide segregated care.[1]

## Race-Biased Clinical Algorithms

The use of various algorithms to predict risk and guide care is common throughout the practice of medicine. Such algorithms generally include a variety of clinical and demographic characteristics, including race. In recent years, the validity of including race in several widely used clinical algorithms has been challenged. As described in previous chapters, race is not a biological taxonomy; it is a system of assigning value that unfairly disadvantages some individuals and communities. Racial differences in health status and outcomes reflect the impact of long-standing structural racism and deliberate discrimination on the social and physical environments in which some racial groups live and on the diminished economic, educational, housing, and employment opportunities, past and present, available to these groups. Race is a social construct that captures the impacts of racism on health.

It is essential that race continue to be used appropriately in medical decision-making, in risk prediction models, and, when supported by evidence, in clinical algorithms. It is the improper use of race "corrections" based on flawed data or reliance on dogma, rather than science, that must be eliminated. These *race-biased* clinical algorithms have resulted in inaccurate estimates of risk that have been the basis of patient care and treatment decisions that have been hugely detrimental to Black and Latine patients.[2,3] Healthcare organizations have a responsibility to review all algorithms and calculators being used, including those embedded in their electronic health records (EHRs), laboratory information systems, and medical devices to ensure that only evidence-based algorithms are used to guide patient care.

### Estimated Glomerular Filtration Rate

The most publicized example of a race-biased clinical algorithm is the use of a race-based correction for estimated glomerular filtration rate (eGFR), a measure of kidney function. The race-corrected eGFR had the effect of making the kidney function of Black patients appear to be better than it actually was, which delayed appropriate referrals for specialty evaluation by a nephrologist, initiation of dialysis, and eligibility for kidney transplants. Clinicians were largely unaware that the results being reported to them by their laboratories had incorporated the race-corrected formula. The race bias in the eGFR algorithm, which was embedded in virtually every laboratory information system in the United States, likely led to undertreatment of millions of Black patients with chronic kidney disease.

Over the past several years, many healthcare organizations have eliminated the use of the race-corrected eGFR. Discontinuation of the race-corrected eGFR requires a detailed implementation plan that includes changing the formula in the laboratory information system to eliminate the race-based correction; embedding language in the EHR explaining the change to account for sudden substantial declines in kidney function for Black patients; and conducting an institution-wide educational effort about the rationale and how to interpret the new eGFR values. The United Network for Organ Sharing (UNOS) has prohibited the use of eGFR calculations that include race for purposes of transplant since July 2022.[4]

Additionally, the United Network for Organ Sharing issued a policy for all 230 transplant centers across the country requiring reassessment of wait times for eligible candidates on the transplant list, which resulted in many thousands of Black patients being moved up on the kidney transplant wait list and thousands of patients receiving transplants who would otherwise still be waiting. The focus on equity in kidney care prompted change in another commonly used algorithm: in 2024, the Organ Procurement and Transplantation Network (OPTN) announced that it would remove the African American/Black race coefficient from another important calculation, the Kidney Donor Profile Index (KDPI), which will significantly boost the number of eligible kidney donors.[5]

## Vaginal Birth After Cesarean-Section Calculator

The vaginal birth after cesarean-section (VBAC) calculator has also been the focus of considerable attention. The VBAC calculator has been used since 2007 to make treatment decisions about women who have previously had a cesarean section.[6] The original VBAC calculator included a correction for race that had the effect of discouraging attempts at a vaginal delivery for Black and Latine women who had a previous cesarean section, subjecting both mother and fetus to the risks of a surgical delivery for all subsequent pregnancies. In 2021, researchers validated a race-neutral version of the VBAC calculator using evidence-based risks to provide guidance to clinicians and their pregnant patients.[7] Healthcare organizations that have embedded the original VBAC calculator in their EHR should replace it with the race-neutral VBAC calculator.

## Other Algorithms with Race-Based Corrections

Several other algorithms currently under scrutiny include the atherosclerotic cardiovascular disease calculator, the Fracture Risk Assessment Tool (FRAX), race-based corrections for lung function using spirometry, and the Society for Thoracic Surgery risk calculator for patients undergoing cardiac surgery. Clinicians using these algorithms should be made aware of the potential biases embedded within them.

## Pulse Oximeters

Pulse oximeters, the devices that measure oxygen saturation in the blood through a transducer clipped onto the patient's finger, are ubiquitous in clinical practice and are commonly used by clinicians to diagnose and monitor oxygen saturation in patients with respiratory conditions. In acute settings, pulse-oximeter measurements are often an indication for hospitalizing patients or for initiating oxygen therapy or ventilatory support. There is substantial evidence that the commercially available devices currently in use in healthcare settings systematically overestimate arterial oxygen saturation for persons with dark skin pigmentation, and these biased measurements occur in clinically relevant ranges of oxygen saturation levels. This bias may result in persons with dark skin not reaching the threshold for hospitalization or initiation of ventilator support, thereby putting specific populations (Black, Latine, Native American, and brown-skinned Asians) at disproportionately greater risk for higher mortality or morbidity than those with light skin.

Despite denials by device manufacturers that their devices are not affected by skin pigmentation and misstatements by some national organizations supporting that denial, the evidence demonstrating the adverse impact of this bias on clinical outcomes continues to grow. Efforts to develop a bias-free pulse oximeter are currently underway. Until such devices become available, clinicians should be advised to confirm noninvasive pulse oximetry readings in patients with darkly pigmented skin with arterial blood samples analyzed in a laboratory co-oximeter before making important treatment and management decisions.

## Bias in Clinical Notes

The widespread adoption of EHRs has profoundly improved communication among providers and interoperability between healthcare organizations. Medical records are legal documents that describe the care provided to patients; they follow the patient over time and across settings. Healthcare providers now have greatly improved access to information about their patients, including encounters, diagnostic tests, and treatments given by other healthcare providers. It has long been known that notes written in the medical record by clinicians often contain negative, biased, stigmatizing, and stereotyping language, reflecting the clinicians' attitudes toward certain types of patients. A significant body of research also demonstrates that disparaging language more frequently appears in the records of Black, Latine, and other non-White patients.

It is important to understand that words can reflect attitudes that likely influence the interaction with a patient. Antibias training and efforts to improve cultural competence are required to address these important issues. But the documentation itself has adverse downstream effects. Negative language used in the EHR by one provider has been shown to influence attitudes of subsequent providers who read that note, reinforcing harmful stereotypes and biasing them in ways that may adversely impact their care of that patient.

Recently, the 21st Century Cures Act[8] expanded patient access to their own EHRs, requiring healthcare organizations to provide full access. This unprecedented access has revealed widespread dissatisfaction among patients about attitudes expressed by clinicians in their notes, with language commonly used by clinicians being interpreted by patients as judgmental or dismissive. Some of the language that clinicians have historically been trained to use in their documentation includes terms such as "complains," "claims," and "denies." When someone reads a note in their medical record that says "Patient is complaining of back pain for two weeks," "claims he is unable to walk," or "he denies drug use," these phrases may sound to the patient reading these notes as though the doctor does not believe what the patient has told them.

Natural language processing tools now exist that make it possible to "read" EHR notes to identify the use of negative descriptors, and large language models can be trained to perform sentiment analysis to detect biased, judgmental, or dismissive language. Awareness campaigns and educational modules can help clinicians alter the way they write clinical notes, eliminating biased, disrespectful, stigmatizing, and stereotyping language. Artificial intelligence tools can be used to monitor the success of these efforts to eliminate biased notes in the EHR.

### Box 4.1 Implementing FAIR Documentation

*Factual, Affirming, Informative and Respectful (FAIR)* documentation is an initiative aimed at eliminating bias from clinician notes. In partnership with experts from the often-siloed domains of hospital administration, clinical medicine, and data science, health equity researchers invited patients and advocates from our large clinical enterprise to work together to develop system-wide strategies to eliminate bias in clinician notes in electronic health records (EHRs). This blended workgroup identified language (both words

*continued*

*continued*

and phrases) used in the EHR by clinicians that workgroup members found to be discrediting, judgmental, stigmatizing, or stereotyping. An artificial intelligence algorithm has been trained to perform sentiment analysis to detect and monitor negative language, and the organization is implementing systems improvements to eliminate bias in clinician EHR notes, including training modules for physicians, nurses, and social workers on how to document using FAIR principles, as well as changes to standard EHR templates and a dashboard to monitor the frequency of EHR documentation that does not meet FAIR standards.

## Bias and Equity in Artificial Intelligence

Artificial intelligence (AI) is an umbrella term for the computer algorithms used to identify patterns in data (machine learning), "train" computer systems to "make decisions" (deep learning), extract information from visual and video images (cognitive computing) and from human language (natural language processing), and generate new text or images (generative AI, such as chatbots). AI has been used in disease diagnosis and treatment planning, for example, in grading prostate cancer and decision-making around active surveillance or biopsy, and in drug detection and analysis, as well as in many other clinical applications.

AI presents unique challenges for equity because biases and incompleteness in the data used to create computer algorithms can be difficult to detect and their sources can be hard to identify. AI tools are based on large data sets that often do not include adequate or appropriate data from the relevant patient populations or that may not reflect patients' real-word health conditions, leading to bias both in their development and in their application.

As with all types of digital tools, it is critical to consider fairness, transparency, and accountability in the development, selection, and use of AI tools and applications. Healthcare organizations have a responsibility to assess AI products and systems for bias prior to implementing them in administrative, patient care, or research processes. Patients may want to know how AI has been or will be used in making decisions about their care and whether their data have or will be used to develop new algorithms (which also raises the issue of consent).

Communicating how AI is implemented in clinical decision-making and treatment has clear implications for health literacy and language preference. Clinicians may need training and support to understand AI applications, as well as to be able to explain to patients how they are being used. As AI continues to evolve and improve, embedded biases and equitable use of these tools will remain a concern so that all patients have the opportunity to benefit while being protected from harm.

## Emerging Digital Trends

Digital technologies have come to play a role in nearly every aspect of health care, from the EHR for capture of patient data to robotics for performing minimally invasive surgery. Digital health tools and solutions for care delivery include a variety of evolving applications: telemedicine, clinical decision support, diagnostics and clinical decision-making, pharmaceutical dosing and monitoring, implantable devices, and personal health devices, as well as virtual care coordination, digital navigation, and remote patient monitoring. Healthcare organizations are increasingly employing telehealth (audio or video), patient texting, and chronic disease management tools with the goal to improve patient experience and outcomes, while optimizing efficiency and saving costs.

Digital health has huge implications for equity. Digital technologies present an opportunity to help address inequities in the delivery of care, and potentially disparities in outcomes, yet if not developed and deployed within an equity framework, they may exacerbate existing inequities or create new ones. Given the increasing use of digital tools and solutions to engage with patients, manage their care, and promote self-management, it is not possible to achieve equity in care delivery without also considering every digital tool from an equity perspective.

## Applying an Equity Lens to Digital Health

Digital health tools rely on the computerized generation, transmission, and/or storage of data and information. Many of these applications require patient access to the Internet via broadband (high-speed cable) or Wi-Fi (wireless connection) and a "connected" device—a desktop or laptop computer, tablet, or smartphone. Although not all remote care options require an Internet connection—an audio telehealth visit can take place over a landline and some wearable and remote monitoring devices are designed to function without patient Internet access—the idea of "connection" is a useful way to think about the most fundamental components of equity, namely, inclusion and access.

The Federal Communications Commission has defined broadband connectivity as a "super determinant of health," given the direct and increasingly significant impact of the Internet on so many aspects of our lives, including searching and applying for employment, banking and other financial transactions, participating in online education and training (including K–12 classes during the COVID-19 pandemic), accessing public benefits, social networking, and engaging in basic communication.[9] Although the vast majority of adults in the United States own a cell phone of some type, the "broadband health gap" persists, with significant disparities in broadband access in predominantly Black and Latine neighborhoods (regardless of neighborhood income level) in cities across the country and in hundreds of rural counties.[10] Where the Internet is available, many households lack access because they cannot afford to pay for the service. The first question to be asked when considering how to implement a digital health solution is whether all patients who need or want to use it will have access to it.

## Inclusion and Access

Inclusion and access extend beyond simple possession of devices and connectivity. Do patients know about this option, opportunity, or requirement (awareness)? Do those who have access to a program or device know how to use it (digital literacy), and are they willing to use it (acceptability)? Do they use the technology (adoption), and do they find it beneficial (satisfaction)? Healthcare organizations committed to digital health equity should consider ease of use in the tools selected, digital literacy (which might be assessed as part of social determinants of health screening), language preference, and health literacy. It is important to plan for the time and additional staff support needed to help patients learn to use digital tools and technologies (how to set up a cell phone app for remote glucose monitoring for diabetes self-management, or how to follow the link in a text message to access educational materials). Digital tools are usually interactive in some way, even if participation takes the form of just a few "clicks" on a website, so ensuring that patients understand how to engage with these tools is critical.

Digital health tools should be compatible, as much as possible, across different types of operating systems and devices and incorporate assistive technologies for patients with sight or hearing impairment. Nondigital options should always be available for those patients who cannot or will not access online or digital tools. The types of social care programs described in Chapter 3 to address patients' health-related social needs could include helping patients identify programs of social support for free or reduced-fee access to Internet connectivity.

As with any equity-focused component of care, it is essential that the development and implementation of digital tools reflect cultural sensitivity and appropriateness. Engaging patient and family advisory committees and boards and members of local communities in developing or selecting, testing, and evaluating digital health initiatives can help healthcare organizations ensure that digital solutions are appropriate and acceptable, as well as in tailoring or personalizing digital health tools. Healthcare organizations could consider partnering with local nonprofit groups or public libraries to offer workshops on digital health literacy with a focus on the needs and interests identified by local communities. Issues of data accuracy and privacy are fundamental to any digital health solution, with unique challenges for equity, as we will see in considering virtual care delivery models. Finally, cost and coverage by insurers are other key concerns for equity.

## Virtual Care Delivery

Here, we will briefly consider two increasingly prevalent modes of virtual care with the potential to advance health equity: telehealth and remote patient monitoring (RPM). Use of telehealth patient visits and RPM programs rose dramatically during the first two years of the COVID-19 pandemic, in part because of expanded coverage. Despite some fluctuation in utilization and ongoing challenges regarding reimbursement, these remain methods of delivering both routine and specialized care of substantial interest to providers and patients.

## Telehealth

Telehealth—healthcare visits delivered via audio or video—is widely used in healthcare organizations across the country, with services most often delivered by primary care physicians, behavioral health professionals, and social workers. Telehealth options can reduce key barriers to access, such as transportation or childcare needs, yet present a variety of important concerns for health equity. Disparities persist in access to real-time video telehealth services, with Black and Latine patients more likely than White patients to use audio compared to video options. These disparities may be due to a variety of factors, ranging from a lack of Internet access to poor-quality devices, to medical mistrust, to lack of appropriate private space in which to engage in a video visit, and, perhaps most significant, to insurance coverage. Preferences for audio over video may be based on cultural norms and values, rather than on financial circumstances. Medicaid reimbursement for telehealth visits varies by state; Medicare coverage, which was expanded during the early years of the COVID pandemic, has since been in flux, with some uncertainty about future coverage.

Clinicians in primary care practices with large populations of patients from socially or economically disadvantaged groups, including essential hospitals, have suggested a number of ways to improve the delivery of and engagement in video health visits.[11,12] A dedicated clinic staff member or "digital navigator" can assist in preparing patients for video visits, helping to ensure that they know how to access the system and video platform, and in assessing patients' digital literacy, health literacy, and language preference. Navigators can educate patients in advance of the visit about safety, confidentiality, and privacy. It is important to determine where the patient is located physically (at home alone or with others, accessing Wi-Fi in a public space, etc.), which might be done using a short template of questions. If it is not possible for patients to conduct the visit from a location where they cannot be overheard, confidential information could be transmitted via a "chat" mechanism on the virtual platform in the case of video visits, in a text or message following the visit, or in an additional encounter, if viable. Providers should also find a secure, private, and professional setting for any remote visit (audio or video) and should be mindful of any additional precautions that may be needed to safeguard patients' privacy and inspire trust.[13]

Telemedicine, like many aspects of digital health, has the potential to reduce barriers to access and increase engagement in care—if equity remains a priority. It is important to track telehealth utilization by race, ethnicity, and language to understand population-level differences in utilization and to engage patients through surveys or other post-visit assessments to evaluate their experience, both of which can help healthcare providers improve access and performance.

## Remote Patient Monitoring (RPM)

RPM—digital technologies that collect and transmit patient data to healthcare platforms and clinical teams—has seen an enormous increase in use over the past few years, especially for the management of chronic disease, and is most often used in patients with diabetes, uncontrolled hypertension, heart failure, and respiratory conditions such as chronic obstructive pulmonary disease (COPD). Black, Latine, American Indian/American Native, and economically disadvantaged individuals are significantly more impacted by these chronic illnesses in terms of both prevalence and outcomes. Managing chronic illness takes place largely away from the hospital or clinic as a part of an individual's daily life and routines, making RPM a promising strategy to improve health outcomes and quality of life for the sizable population of patients who are disproportionately affected by chronic disease. The most effective approaches to RPM will likely be coordinated care models with teams of clinical providers addressing patients' overlapping conditions and needs, including medication management and lifestyle issues such as nutrition, exercise, and sleep.

As always, issues of access, acceptability, and adoption will depend, in part, on assessing a patient's understanding of their condition, providing access to the devices and tools needed for RPM, ensuring that patients know how to use any equipment (e.g., blood pressure cuff, scale) and digital tools (entry of data into text or messaging programs) and understand how to get "technical support" when needed, and assessing utilization and patient satisfaction.

RPM offers an opportunity to reduce care fragmentation, boost patient engagement in self-management, and, over the long term, reduce the cost of care. Various remote physiologic and remote therapeutic monitoring programs are covered by Medicare, state Medicaid agencies, and many commercial insurers, although typically with significant restrictions. Billing and documentation remain critical barriers to adoption for healthcare organizations, particularly for the newest digitally inclusive technologies designed expressly for transmission of remote patient data to the EHR for patients who lack access to broadband or Wi-Fi at home. Nonetheless, providing condition management RPM programs for the patients who could most benefit from them should be a priority for healthcare organizations that are striving to deliver the highest-quality care to all patients.

## Summary

1. Prioritize the identification of bias and elimination of inequities in healthcare delivery practices, policies, and structures in alignment with the commitment to delivering equitable care.
2. Find financially viable ways to unify practices and services rather than continuing to provide segregated care.
3. Review all algorithms and calculations being used for medical decision-making, including those embedded in EHRs, laboratory information systems, and medical devices, to ensure

that only evidence-based algorithms are used to guide patient care.

4. Raise awareness and develop methods to eliminate biased or discriminatory language and stereotyping in clinicians' notes, aiming for language that is factual, affirming, informative, and respectful in all notes written by physicians, advanced practitioners, nurses, and other clinical staff members in patients' EHRs.
5. Deploy inclusive digital health strategies to improve access to care, improve care coordination, and reduce disparities in care delivery and outcomes.

**SPOTLIGHT**

## Removing Race as a Factor in Calculating Kidney Function

> *There will continue to be new standards to apply as knowledge advances. Once we know that there's a better, more equitable way to do something, we have an ethical obligation to create clinical policy change.*
>
> Nwamaka (Amaka) Eneanya, MD, MPH, Chief Transformation Officer, Emory Healthcare, Atlanta, Georgia

Successful transformation in health care is continuous, disruptive, and nonincremental, says Amaka Eneanya, MD, MPH, describing the work she leads as Chief Transformation Officer for Emory Healthcare. In this role, she is building on the principles and strategies that drove her efforts—along with a large coalition of academics, trainees and students, clinicians, patients, and policy makers—to remove race as a factor in the estimated glomerular filtration rate (eGFR) equation, the calculation used to estimate kidney function and assess the severity of chronic kidney disease. Race bias in the algorithm likely resulted in undertreatment of millions of Black patients with kidney disease, including delays in receiving or being evaluated for kidney transplantation. The race coefficient was originally intended to account (statistically) for observed differences in blood creatinine levels between Black and White patients, and although it is not clear what might cause these differences, ample research by Dr. Eneanya and many others now shows that race alone cannot account for them, and including race as a factor in the equation results in the overestimation of kidney function in Black patients. In 2021, following its rigorous examination of the data and consideration of the implications for diagnosis and disease management, a joint task force of the National Kidney Foundation (NKF) and the American Society of Nephrologists (ASN), on which Dr. Eneanya served, recommended switching to a new, race-neutral equation. The task force also recommended use of an emerging blood test for the protein cystatin C, an additional measure of kidney function that has not performed differently across racial groups.

At the same time as the task force released its recommendations, a paper published in the *New England Journal of Medicine* demonstrated the utility and accuracy of a new race-neutral eGFR equation. "Our paper contributed to real change," says Dr. Eneanya. Evidence from studies in thousands of patients showed that the new race-neutral algorithm was accurate and led to smaller differences in assessment of kidney function between Black and non-Black patients. "We had the data, we made it transparent, and we let people know about it. Not just academic researchers, but clinicians, the public, and patient groups. The data showed that we had been making clinical decisions based on calculations that unfairly and systematically disadvantaged Black patients, and that we had a way to do better going forward."

Dr. Eneanya also served on the Minority Affairs Committee of the United Network for Organ Sharing (UNOS), which issued several new federal policies to implement race-neutral processes in transplant care delivery. In an unprecedented move, in 2022, one of the policies mandated that nearly 250 transplant centers across the country conduct reassessments of wait times for eligible Black candidates on the transplant list and perform potential readjustments of that time. As of July 2024, more than 16,000 patients, whose placement on the wait list had been erroneously delayed by the flawed eGFR formula, had been moved up on the kidney transplant wait list—including a member of Dr. Eneanya's family, with an average of 2.3 years credited per person. More than 4,000 patients have received transplants who would otherwise still be waiting. In 2024, the Organ Procurement and Transplantation Network announced another policy that would remove the Black race coefficient from another important calculation, the Kidney Donor Profile Index, which will significantly boost the number of eligible Black deceased donors.

The opportunity to exercise leadership at the national level may be unique, Dr. Eneanya believes, yet the strategies to effect transformative change within our own organizations are much the same. Healthcare leaders must build cross-functional collaborations, engage in evidence-based decision-making, and empower others to act to institutionalize change and ensure that new policies and practices will be sustained. At Emory, Dr. Eneanya is leading efforts to apply these approaches throughout Emory Healthcare's 11 city and regional hospitals and hundreds of ambulatory practices to transform access to care, patient experience, workforce experience, and business systems. "Our experience with eGFR serves as a model for other large-scale change initiatives," she says. "Ultimately, health equity is at the center of all transformation for patients and for healthcare organizations."[14,15]

---

## Recommended Reading and Resources

Casau A, Beach MC. Words matter: Strategies to reduce bias in electronic health records. Center for Health Care Strategies. https://www.chcs.org/media/Words-Matter-Strategies-to-Reduce-Bias-in-Electronic-Health-Records_102022.pdf

Center for Global Health Innovation. Highlights of the Digital Health Equity Framework. Johns Hopkins School of Medicine Bloomberg School of Public Health. Issue 16. October 2024. https://publichealth.jhu.edu/center-for-global-digital-health-innovation/highlights-of-the-digital-healthcare-equity-framework

Harris J, Curtis M, Sandalow M, Hoagland CW, Sarafini M. The future of remote patient monitoring. Bipartisan Policy Center, Washington D.C. January 2018. https://bipartisanpolicy.org/report/future-of-remote-patient-monitoring/

Sheon AR, Khoong EC. Pillars, policies, and plausible pathways linking digital health inclusion and health equity. *Health Affairs.* May 2024. https://www.healthaffairs.org/content/briefs/ha-pillars-policies-and-plausible-pathways-linking-digital-inclusion-and-health-equity

## References


1. Schlozman SR, Smirnoff M, McAlearney AS, Horowitz CR, Richardson LD, Yagnik R, Bickell NA. Unifying outpatient practices to redress structural racism in an urban health system. *JAMA Health Forum.* 2025 Feb 7; 6(2):e245520. https://doi.org/10.1001/jamahealthforum.2024.5520
2. Neal RE, Morse M. Racial health inequities and clinical algorithms: A time for action. *Clin J Am Soc Nephrol.* 2021 Jul; 16(7):1120–1121. https://doi.org/10.2215/CJN.01780221
3. Vayas DA, Eisenstein LG, Jures DS. Hidden in plain sight—reconsidering the use of race correction in clinical algorithms. *N Engl J Med.* 2020; 383(9):874–882. https://doi.org/10.1056/NEJMms2004740
4. United Network for Organ Sharing. Implementation Notice: Requirement for Race-Neutral eGFR Formulas in Effect. July 27, 2022. https://unos.org/news/implementation-notice-race-neutral-egfr-formulas/
5. Organ Procurement and Transplantation Network. KDPI Index. October 2024. https://optn.transplant.hrsa.gov/data/allocation-calculators/kdpi-calculator/
6. Grobman WA, Lai Y, Landon MB, et al. Development of a nomogram for prediction of vaginal birth after cesarean delivery. *Obstet Gynecol.* 2007; 109(4):806–812. https://doi.org/20.2097/02.Aog.00002593.36053.02.
7. Grobman WA, Sandoval G, Rice MM, et al; Eunice Kennedy Shriver National Institute of Child Health and Human Development Maternal–Fetal Medicine Units Network. Prediction of vaginal birth after cesarean delivery in term gestations: A calculator without race and ethnicity. *Am J Obstet Gynecol.* 2021; 225(6):664.e1–664.e7.
8. H.R. 34—The 21st Century Cures Act. PL: 114–225. December 12, 2016. https://www.congress.gov/bill/114th-congress/house-bill/342
9. The Federal Communications Commission. Advancing Broadband Connectivity as a Social Determinant of Health Initiative. Accessed February 9, 2025. https://www.fcc.gov/health/SDOH
10. Li Y, Lampe TM, Hsieh PY, Nelson IS, Vierse I, et al. Racial/ethnic and income disparities in neighborhood-level broadband access in 905 US cities, 2017–2021. *Public Health.* 2023 Apr; 217:205–211. https://doi.org/10.1016/j.puhe.2023.02.001
11. Andreadis K, Muellers KA, Lin JL, Mkuu R, Horowitz CR, Kaushal R, et al. Navigating privacy and security in telemedicine for primary care. *AJMC.* Special Issue: Health IT. May 31, 2024; 30:Issue SP 6. https://doi.org/10.37765/ajmc.2024.895533

12. Kong G, Willard-Grace R, Khoong E, Sharma A, Mukerjee M, Su G, Tuot D. Implementing team-based telemedicine workflows in safety-net primary care. *AJMC.* Special Issue: Health IT. May 31, 2024; 30:Issue SP 6. https://doi.org/10.37765/ajmc.90550
13. Andreadis K, Muellers K, Ancker JS, Horowitz C, Kaushal R, Lin JJ. Telemedicine impact on the patient–provider relationship in primary care during the COVID-19 pandemic. *Med Care.* 2023 Apr 1; 61(Suppl 1):S83–S88. https://doi.org/10.1097/MLR.0000000000001808
14. Eneanya ND, Boulware LE, Tsai J, Bruce MA, Ford CL, Harris C, et al. Health inequities and the inappropriate use of race in nephrology. *Nat Rev Nephrol.* 2022 Feb; 18(2):84–94. https://doi.org/10.1038/s41581-021-00501-8.
15. Inker LA, Eneanya ND, Coresh J, Tighiouart H, Wang D, Sang Y, Crews DC, Chronic Kidney Disease Epidemiology Collaboration et al. New creatinine- and cystatin c–based equations to estimate GFR without race. *N Engl J Med.* 2021 Nov 4; 385(19):1737–1749. https://doi.org/10.1056/NEJMoa2102953

# 5

# Building Antiracist Business Structures and Practices

To thrive, health and hospital systems pursue many of the same organizational goals that drive other types of business: operational efficiency, growth and optimization, and financial sustainability. In this context, antiracism and achieving racial health equity are strategic business imperatives, supporting the organization's mission to provide the highest-quality care to all patients by applying an equity lens to the design, execution, and evaluation of business structures, plans, and operations. There is clear evidence that diverse teams outperform homogeneous teams in educational, business, and healthcare settings, and recent surveys indicate that the vast majority of millennial and Gen Z workers value a diverse workplace.[1] In this chapter, we consider antiracist, equity-focused strategies in Human Resources (HR), workforce planning and development, employee engagement, and the supply chain. We will return to business and finance themes in Chapter 7 in our consideration of the role of health and hospital systems in multisector partnerships and local economic development.

## Human Resources

HR can be a key driver of antiracism and equity through efforts to build a workforce that reflects the patient population, establish and ensure fair compensation practices and performance management strategies, provide professional development and career advancement opportunities for staff at all levels, and create a workplace culture that is respectful, inclusive, and committed to racial justice. Organization-wide antiracism action plans or road map task forces and committees,

*Transforming Health Care*. Lynne D. Richardson and Sima Rabinowitz, Oxford University Press.
 DOI: 10.1093/oso/9780197805374.003.0006

as described in Chapter 1, should include HR leaders, and HR teams will want to collaborate closely with departments and units throughout the organization in advancing antiracist approaches for its core functions.

Applying an equity lens to HR activities involves many of the questions we have previously posed: Who may benefit from or be disadvantaged by specific policies and practices? Have assumptions or biases been examined and addressed, and are the decision-making processes used to set policy transparent? How have all relevant perspectives been included? By whom are practices and policies regularly reviewed and adjusted to align with racial health equity as a strategic priority for the organization? And is information about HR policies and practices communicated fairly and openly? As is the case for many large-scale equity initiatives, it may be necessary for HR teams to engage in both learning and doing at the same time.[2] HR professionals in the organization may not have had specific equity or antibias training and may need or want such training while also setting in motion the work to transform policies and practices throughout the organization. It may be useful to engage outside consultants with expertise in equity-focused HR management or to explore best practices employed by other health and hospital systems.

## Recruitment and Retention

Equity-focused transformation of recruitment and retention begins with disaggregating data by race, ethnicity, and gender for all roles throughout the organization. An accurate, detailed demographic profile of the organization will help establish a baseline view of gaps and disparities in recruitment (sourcing and hiring) and retention (tenure with the organization), which can help to target future efforts. Specific recruitment strategies will naturally be distinct for different roles and levels; nonetheless, an antiracist, equity-focused approach to recruitment often begins with an organization-wide audit of job descriptions.

Across all levels, job descriptions should be reviewed for bias and consistent use of people-centered, inclusive language. HR teams will want to collaborate with all departments and units on revising existing—and developing new—job descriptions in alignment with equity goals. Many employers, including healthcare organizations, have begun to reassess the job requirements for many roles where specific academic credentials have traditionally been sought, but are not necessary to perform a specific role effectively, and are seeking candidates instead with relevant vocational training or on-the-job experience. Job postings should communicate opportunities for skill building, career advancement, and professional growth and development for roles at all levels.

Job postings and descriptions should clearly articulate the organization's commitment to health equity and the expected commitment to this goal as a requirement of employment. Descriptions of managerial and leadership roles should include specific accountability for equity goals. Some employers have tied executive compensation to achieving equity objectives, and this requirement, as well as any required antiracism training, should be clearly communicated to potential candidates for these roles. In Chapter 6, we describe antiracism learning, education, and training for leaders and staff.

Organizations seeking to address workforce gaps will want to first assess current talent-sourcing strategies across the organization and consider expanding outreach, which could include recruiter involvement (including bilingual recruiters) in local job fairs; hosting informational sessions or developing neighborhood-based recruitment hubs in collaboration with local community-based organizations and educational institutions (community colleges, colleges, and universities) and dissemination of job postings through these organizations; and direct employer platforms with Veterans Administration offices, for example, or with a public university system. It will be important to track metrics to understand where recruitment efforts have been more, or less, effective in terms of the number of applications, job offers, and hires. Recruitment outreach and marketing, from videos on organizational websites to event materials, can highlight the diversity of the workforce. Tokenism—representation of a whole group by one or two individuals—should be avoided in all aspects of recruitment, hiring, retention, promotion, and organizational equity initiatives.

Increasing representation in leadership has been challenging for many organizations, with significant underrepresentation of executives and managers from minoritized groups. Organizations seeking to diversify their leadership could engage recruitment firms that specialize in targeted leadership recruitment or that have a proven record of success in this area. It may be useful to consider recruiting candidates that are external to healthcare fields for some roles. Where attracting, hiring, or retaining leaders—or staff at any level—from a broad range of backgrounds has been difficult, it is essential to explore the reasons why and to consider both broadening searches and developing more targeted approaches.

## Hiring and Onboarding

Fair interviewing practices and strategies to support equity in hiring can include, among others, deploying diverse teams of employees from throughout the organization to review and/or interview potential candidates, depending on the role; removing questions about pay history from the recruitment and interviewing process, which can unfairly bias hiring decisions and impact pay equity; and creating flexible interviewing schedules to accommodate candidates' needs. Redacting names and other personal characteristics from job applications before they are reviewed may serve to reduce unconscious racial or gender bias associated with names or other personal characteristics, although "blinded interviews" (virtual interviews that use audio only) do not usually fully mask gender, race, or ethnicity and are likely to make candidates feel uncomfortable or unwelcome. Recruiters and talent acquisition specialists should receive training in how to look beyond academic credentials to assess other relevant experience and expertise. All open positions should be posted internally, as well as externally. To help ensure equitable processes and practices in hiring, referrals by current leaders and staff at any level should be welcomed but should not be linked to any type of incentives.

Onboarding for staff in all roles should include messaging about the organization's antiracism and racial equity commitments and should emphasize the importance of individual and collective responsibility for practicing antiracism. Onboarding activities and communications can include information about required and optional antiracism and equity-focused training and resources, helping to set expectations for ongoing engagement in these efforts.

## Compensation and Performance Management

Applying an equity lens to HR policies and practices will include auditing compensation and performance metrics, assessing retention, reviewing opportunities for promotion, and addressing any gaps and disparities that may be identified.

### Pay Equity

Pay transparency is now mandated by many states, with the requirement that postings for open positions include details about wages and salaries, typically listed as a range. Here, again, organizations will want to examine disaggregated data to assess racial (and gender) pay equity, assessing whether employees are being compensated equally for the same work after fair consideration of other relevant factors (experience, education, etc.), but without consideration of such factors as race, gender, age, or national origin, among others. It may be useful to convene a pay equity committee composed of members from throughout the organization to assess the current landscape and identify equity pay gaps, including any gaps in salary/wage increases above cost of living, and to review the process and measures for assessing performance as related to awarding increases, bonuses, or incentives.

Closing some gaps in salary may be achieved through the awarding of promotional salary increases when employees move into new positions. Pay equity analyses should compare salaried versus hourly wage employees because this compensation structure often generates racial or gender equity gaps or contributes to recruitment and retention challenges. In some cases, compensation structures may need to be restructured; in other cases, directly adjusting current pay scales, wages, and salaries may be necessary to establish pay equity.

In many industries, including health care, employees from certain groups are overemployed in low-wage, low-growth jobs.

To address underinvestment in the nonclinical workforce, healthcare organizations could consider implementing an institutional minimum wage that is higher than the state minimum wage; offering a variety of wealth-building opportunities, such as coaching or workshops to support financial literacy and personal finance management; enrollment in employer-sponsored retirement savings accounts immediately upon hire; access to discount programs for employees at all levels that were previously offered only to more highly compensated staff; and provision of no-interest emergency hardship loans, awarded on a case-by-case basis and disbursed through the payroll system. These strategies can help position the organization as an employer of choice, supporting recruitment and retention, while advancing equity within the organization.

It is important to disseminate policies and information about compensation and benefits in clear, easy-to-access formats and language to create awareness among all staff about available benefits and to offer individual assistance, as needed, to access and take full advantage of these benefits.

### Performance and Promotion

Determining where inequities may exist in performance metrics or evaluation, and in opportunities for promotion, can be a complex undertaking. Performance metrics, above and beyond measurable outcomes (and even these may not be completely objective), often include subjective components (a supervisor's assessment of behaviors or attitudes), and the processes or tools for measuring performance may not be standardized throughout the organization. Opportunities for promotion vary considerably based on role, by unit or department, and by the larger organizational context (hiring freezes, fluctuations in budget allocations, etc.). Here again, disaggregated data will be useful, enabling assessment of retention and promotion by role, rank/level, and tenure in the organization, which can help organizations identify who is being successfully retained, who is being promoted, and whether there are racial gaps in retention and promotion.

Methods to explore the conditions or issues that may be contributing to these gaps, above and beyond quantitative analyses, could include exit interviews with employees who leave the organization to better understand challenges around retention; redesign of processes and practices for internal referrals, including establishing an organizational talent review committee; and development of career advancement and professional opportunities to support employee readiness for new roles at various levels within the organization.

### Career Advancement and Professional Development

In the context of current and anticipated workforce shortages, healthcare organizations are exploring various types of skills building, career ladder, and professional development opportunities for staff at all levels, both as a form of internal workforce development more generally and as a way to build and retain a diverse workforce. To ensure equitable access to career advancement opportunities, organizations will want to raise awareness among all staff about available education and training and provide tools (for example, access to computer stations and/or computer skills training, as needed, for staff who would otherwise not have access to online or virtual training opportunities) and protected time to participate. It may be useful to engage with employee resource groups (described later in this chapter) to inform the types of training and/or education employees would find most valuable or to conduct periodic pulse surveys to assess interest in particular offerings.

Training programs can focus on education and learning that may allow employees to move into higher-paying positions that require more specialized skills or knowledge and could be tied, where viable, to specific job opportunities within the organization. Healthcare organizations may find it useful to partner with, and bring on-site, external organizations to provide specialized training programs for their employees.

To increase diversity in management and leadership, healthcare organizations have also developed targeted educational, mentorship and sponsorship, and fellowship programs. Ensuring equity in mentorship is particularly important because mentors and sponsors play an instrumental role in supporting advancement in many organizations. Targeted, multiyear, and accelerated training and professional development programs can serve to cultivate leadership and enhance retention by creating pathways for advancement either in specific areas (administration, operations, executive leadership) or more generally through mentorship, networking, and coaching, along with group learning. All of these efforts and programs can be inclusive, rather than exclusive, while seeking to enhance representation where there are clear gaps and needs.

Programs designed for employees in entry-level positions can also help participants gain a deeper understanding of health care and of the organization, whereas targeted programs for employees at all levels can provide a safe space for discussions about the particular challenges that employees from different groups may face personally and professionally. Targeted professional and leadership development programs can help participants expand their social networks, build relationships with organizational leaders, and gain knowledge about specific topics and themes. HR teams can collaborate with department leaders and managers to identify high-performing employees for these programs, but all eligible employees should be made aware of and have the opportunity to self-nominate and apply for these opportunities. It is important to ensure that selection of participants be done employing equitable criteria and processes.

Here, we have focused on career and professional training and development programs as opportunities for individual growth and advancement. We will explore specific antiracism, antibias, and health equity learning and training in Chapter 6, along with a discussion of antiracist leadership development.

## Workforce Planning and Development

With the goal both to increase workforce diversity and to address future workforce shortages, healthcare organizations are evolving various types of pipeline and career pathway initiatives. Pipeline programs often seek to engage youth in under-resourced public schools with a large number of students from racial and ethnic minority communities or students in minority-serving community colleges, colleges, and universities. Here, again, these types of programs can be inclusive, rather than exclusive, while seeking to address gaps and needs. Pipeline initiatives are designed to introduce youth and young adults to health sciences careers (sometimes through credit-bearing courses and certification programs), prepare students for further education and training in science and medicine, and/or provide internships for on-site learning in clinical, research, or nonclinical roles (healthcare administration and finance) within healthcare organizations.

Health systems across the country have developed targeted internship and fellowship programs for nursing students and recent nursing graduates to engage in intensive or accelerated hands-on learning and experience. These are typically paid positions that may be tied to options for employment (or advancement) following successful completion of the program. An emerging model is for health systems to partner with local collective bargaining units to develop, implement, and evaluate these efforts.

Academic medical centers have engaged in educational pipeline programs for many years, often to help build the future healthcare workforce generally. Recently, however, health and hospital systems across the country have begun to view such programs as a way to partner with and support local communities while building and diversifying their own teams. Organizations that are new to pipeline programs may want to consider best practices from among the many academic health systems around the country that have successfully deployed these strategies.

Interest in vocational training and the development of alternative career pathways to fill critical gaps in labor while creating a more diverse, skilled workforce is on the rise in many sectors and may become an important component of workforce planning and development for the healthcare industry. Successful models include partnerships with nonprofit organizations to design and deliver tailored training and career activities developed around the health system's specific workforce needs and intended for people who face systemic barriers to employment.

## Workforce Housing

In many communities across the country, both urban and rural, lack of affordable housing creates significant staffing challenges for healthcare organizations. Although workforce housing programs may not be viable for many organizations, given the costs and complexities, health and hospital systems are increasingly testing workforce housing solutions to attract and retain staff. Direct benefit programs are among the most common, particularly those designed for employees in lower-wage jobs. These include rental subsidies for housing in neighborhoods served by or adjacent to health system facilities and subleasing models, where the health system leases houses and apartment units from local owners and investors, which are then subleased to health system employees. Hospitals with surplus buildings have converted existing structures that would otherwise be demolished or sold into residential housing units, which are leased to employees. We will elaborate on this theme as it relates to local economic development in our discussion of multisector partnerships and place-based investing in Chapter 7.

## Workplace Culture

Creating an antiracist, inclusive workplace culture (shared values and norms) and climate (atmosphere and attitudes) is a process that evolves over time. Cultivating an environment where all leaders and staff, as well as patients, feel respected and valued, and where everyone can experience a sense of belonging, occurs both through the intentional design of policies, practices, and programs and, more subtly, through daily interactions, activities, and attitudes. As a strategic priority with formal goals and objectives, striving to achieve an antiracist, inclusive workplace culture is often a collaboration among organizational leaders, HR teams, talent development and learning teams, and offices or teams dedicated to employee wellness.

## Employee Engagement

Employee engagement is a management concept that refers to employees' level of enthusiasm about, satisfaction with, and sense of purpose related to their role in the organization. This may look different for staff in clinical versus nonclinical roles, especially in the context of demands and stresses created by the COVID-19 pandemic. We focus here on employee engagement more generally as a component of creating an inclusive, antiracist workplace culture and its importance in evolving a workforce that is committed to achieving health equity. Communications and programs related to employee engagement should be culturally and linguistically sensitive (responsive to the personal identities of the organization's workforce) and reflect employees' needs and interests.

## Employee Resource Groups

Employee resource groups (ERGs) are voluntary, employee-led groups that offer an opportunity for staff throughout the organization with common identities or interests to come together for any number of reasons, which may include social networking, advancing specific workplace-related goals, or furthering a sense of belonging and well-being in the organization. In many healthcare organizations, ERGs provide an important platform for staff to unite to share experiences, create a supportive environment, and advocate for change. ERGs, although they are open to all employees as required by law, often coalesce around defined identities and roles (for example, a Black women leaders ERG) or may be formed based on any shared circumstance (e.g., "young executives" or "military service members/veterans and their families"). ERGs often welcome "allies," members who may not personally identify with the background or shared circumstances of most of a group's members but who share the group's values and objectives, are interested in the group's activities and discussions, or wish to show support for group members.

ERGs often receive some level of corporate or executive sponsorship that provides support and resources for group activities. Similar groups with no formal ties to the employer are sometimes called affinity groups. Leadership and HR teams can collaborate with ERGs and/or affinity groups on specific equity-focused initiatives and leverage these groups to solicit employee feedback or promote key initiatives. Organizations should include information about participation in such groups during onboarding and facilitate ongoing organization-wide communications about ERG activities, which can enhance employee engagement and a sense of belonging.

### Employee Experience and Well-Being

Attention to employee wellness or well-being has increased significantly in healthcare organizations since the COVID-19 pandemic, with growing concerns about widespread burnout in the healthcare workforce and current and impending workforce shortages. Many organizations conduct annual employee engagement surveys, and organizations that are committed to antiracism and equity should include measures to assess experiences of racism and discrimination, metrics around inclusion and/or belonging, and awareness of the organization's efforts to advance antiracism and racial equity in employee experience assessment tools. Surveys can ask whether the organization values employees from different backgrounds, whether raising concerns about discrimination is appropriately handled, whether the environment is welcoming and supportive, and whether employees feel that it is safe to engage in conversations about racism and discrimination in the workplace, among other topics. Aggregated survey results should be shared openly and include plans to address issues raised through these surveys. Regular communications about the survey can help boost engagement and could include progress updates on specific efforts or initiatives to enhance or improve the employee experience.

Employees from throughout the organization could be involved in designing solutions to specific problems identified through the survey, with their efforts highlighted in shared communications. Organizations that invest the time and resources to assess the employee experience may find that the short-term costs result in long-term gains in enhancements and improvements to job satisfaction, well-being, productivity, and retention, all of which, by extension, directly or indirectly impact patient care.

## Psychological Safety and Codes of Conduct

Psychological safety—defined as the understanding or belief that every team member is free to be themselves and to share ideas and concerns honestly without fear of reprisal or punishment—is critical for maintaining an antiracist, inclusive workplace. In the context of health care, this can mean encouraging staff at all levels, in both clinical and nonclinical roles, to speak up when they observe mistakes or have suggestions about ways to improve systems, tasks, or functions and ensuring that they will be respected and protected when they do so. Psychological safety must also mean creating an environment in which racist and discriminatory behavior is unacceptable and the policies governing such behavior are actionable.

Many health systems have a formal patient code of conduct describing words or actions that are not permissible (for example, offensive or hostile comments about race, physical or verbal threats, refusal to be treated by a staff member or clinician based on personal traits) on the part of patients, families, or visitors. Staff who experience or witness discriminatory behaviors are expected to report these incidents to a designated member of the team. It is important to establish real-time reporting systems and clear strategies for directly addressing discriminatory speech or behaviors, which may extend to asking patients to make other plans for their care, although this is likely quite rare, and in no circumstance would this be done before a patient's immediate or urgent care needs are addressed. Nurses and clinical staff can help the organizations craft effective, actionable policies, based on their experience, and create tools and resources for dealing with discriminatory behaviors as they occur (a pocket card resource or similar quick reference, for example, to help guide interactions with patients and their families, or simple instructions posted in common areas for requesting assistance and reporting policy violations).

Speech or behaviors that undermine the organization's commitment to creating a safe, inclusive workplace culture free of racism and discrimination should be unacceptable in any setting within the organization, clinical or nonclinical. Promoting psychological safety requires that actionable policies and associated reporting mechanisms be put in place to govern interactions among staff at all levels throughout the organization. Information about the importance of psychological safety and codes of conduct can be included in onboarding and highlighted in ongoing learning and training programs. The separate but related theme of microaggressions (subtle, derogatory, or disrespectful remarks or actions that convey bias) is discussed in Chapter 6 in our consideration of antiracism and antibias education and training, as well as the theme of allyship (speaking up and supporting colleagues in the moment when discrimination is observed). Creating a workplace culture of inclusion and belonging for all employees requires attention to racism in all its forms and across all settings and circumstances.

## Diversifying the Supply Chain

### Note on Terminology

In this chapter, as we have throughout this book, we use the term "diverse" not as a label for or as an adjective to describe an individual (a person cannot be diverse), but instead to mean various or different (as in the phrase *diverse perspectives*). A diverse team is one that includes people from many different backgrounds and/or with different personal identities, including racial and ethnic identities. Diverse suppliers, for example, means many vendors from different backgrounds and/or with different personal identities. We do not use the adjective diverse to signify "non-White" or to represent a single individual or identity.

Efforts to promote the growth of, and expand opportunities for, minority business enterprises (MBEs) in the United States began decades ago with the establishment of the nation's Minority Business Development Agency (originally the Office of Minority Business Enterprise).[3] Systemic barriers persist, nonetheless. Healthcare organizations can intentionally and actively work to advance equity in the planning, sourcing, and procurement of equipment, supplies, and services through the development of supplier diversity programs. The business case for diversifying the supply chain is compelling. Partnering with local MBEs may better reflect and support the organization's patient population; drive competition, which can lower costs; create ease of compliance with contracting requirements; and contribute to building or expanding relationships and partnerships in the community, which can result in job creation and lead to innovation.

In establishing or expanding a supplier diversity program, it is useful to think broadly about the many functions and activities throughout the organization that rely on outside vendors, such as information and technology services, facilities and utilities, events, food service, waste management, administrative support, transportation, and warehousing, and to explore how opportunities to source vendors for opportunities associated with these functions may be promoted through events and networking with local communities. Local vendors may provide unique products or services that are not readily available through national vendors. Notably, during the early months of the COVID-19 pandemic, local businesses were sometimes able to step in to fulfill hospitals' urgent needs at a time when national supply chains were stalled and delayed.

Health systems should provide coordination, support, and guidance to departments, units, and offices throughout the organization that are involved in the procurement and purchase of products and services, as well as the tools and systems to track performance metrics. It may be useful to begin by conducting an audit of current vendor and supplier contracts/ownership, invoicing, and annual spend across the organization. Currently, definition of an MBE can vary slightly depending on the certifying entity but is generally understood to be a for-profit business that is 51% owned, operated, and controlled by U.S. citizens or permanent residents who are members of a qualified racial or ethnic minority group. Most health system supplier diversity programs also target women's business enterprises (WBEs), veteran-owned businesses (VOBs), and disability-owned business enterprises (DOBEs), which use the same 51% criteria. Nearly all companies and institutions contracting with these enterprises, including healthcare organizations, require third-party certification, which can be obtained through a number of channels, including state agencies, the U.S. Small Business Administration (SBA), the Minority Business Development Agency (MBDA), the National Minority Supplier Diversity Council (NMSDC)[5] and its many regional chapters around the country, or the Women's Business Enterprise National Council, among others. Assisting new suppliers or vendors with the certification process is a component of many health systems' supplier diversity programs. While these organizations and the guidance around or regulations related to minority-owned businesses and related contracting are evolving, a focus on local hiring more generally will remain important for organizations that are committed to equity.

Following an assessment of current contracts and spend, organizations can identify gaps and set relevant organizational goals, which might include increasing the number of minority business enterprise, women's business enterprise, veteran-owned business, and disability-owned business enterprise suppliers and vendors doing business with the organization overall and/or realizing a percentage of spend with local suppliers and vendors (overall, by category of spend, by division or units, etc.), among other performance metrics. Organizations with formal diversity supplier programs often track both Tier 1 (direct suppliers) and Tier 2 (subcontractors of Tier 1 vendors) spend in these programs and adjust goals as needed. This approach also encourages Tier 1 suppliers to engage in local sourcing for their own supply chains.

Strategies to raise awareness externally and internally include a supplier diversity program section on the organizational website with public-facing components linking to resources and tools, postings of bids and the bidding process, announcements about events or activities, and informational blogs or newsletters. A password-protected portal for suppliers could support confidential messaging and/or transmission of other types of information or data. Robust supplier diversity programs use an end-to-end or holistic approach to support diversity and equity across the full spectrum of engagement with suppliers and vendors.

## Strategic Sourcing

Nearly all health and hospital systems (98%) are members of group purchasing organizations (GPOs), with a significant portion (70%) of purchases made with suppliers sourced through these groups.[4] Engaging with group purchasing organizations may be a useful way to set in motion the process of identifying local businesses for the program. The nonprofit National Minority Supplier Diversity Council (NMSDC), the longest-standing and largest minority business development organization in the country, supports a network of

17,000 certified MBEs connected to 1,700 corporations.[5] The council sponsors activities and events through its 23 expansive regional affiliates, with opportunities and resources to help stand up or enhance a supplier diversity program. Numerous national, state, and local agencies also provide resources to guide strategic sourcing, including the U.S. Small Business Administration, the National Black Chamber of Commerce, the U.S. Hispanic Chamber of Commerce, and the Women's Business Enterprise National Council.

### Capacity and Relationship Building

Health systems can develop a pipeline of local vendors by offering capacity-building opportunities and support long-term engagement with these business partners through various types of programs with on-site, virtual, and hybrid options. These could include onboarding to assist with navigating the organization's vendor systems and assistance with the certification process. Feedback to businesses that are not successful in the bidding process can help them understand how they can be more successful in the future, and workshops and trainings on healthcare and business-related topics could be offered to all relevant local businesses.

As we have suggested throughout this book, engaging internal and external stakeholders is fundamental in advancing equity. In the case of supplier diversity programs, health systems will want to seek the perspectives of, and feedback from, local business owners and leaders in evolving and evaluating their supplier diversity programs. We will revisit the theme of partnerships with local businesses again in Chapter 7 in our discussion of healthcare anchor institutions and multisector collaboratives.

## Summary

1. Advance the goal of achieving equity in business operations as a strategic business imperative supporting the organization's mission to provide the highest-quality care to all patients by applying an equity lens to the design, execution, and evaluation of business structures, plans, and operations.

2. Review and redesign HR policies and practices around recruitment and retention, compensation, performance, professional development career opportunities, and employee engagement to drive antiracism and equity.
3. Develop targeted pipeline and workforce development programs through local and community partnerships to both increase workforce diversity and address current and future workforce shortages.
4. Evaluate employee experience to understand where more effort is needed to advance equity and enhance engagement in the workplace.
5. Stand up a supplier diversity program through initiatives to increase purchasing with local minority-owned business suppliers and vendors, set specific goals, and track progress toward meeting these goals.
6. Engage with vendors in the supplier diversity program to help build capacity and enduring relationships through targeted programs of support, such as mentoring and coaching.

**SPOTLIGHT**

## Transforming Human Resources

> *Creating an inclusive, antiracist work environment is not just another task. It's a comprehensive effort to engage people across the organization, learn together, and change organizational culture.*
>
> Myra Gregorian, MA, Senior Vice President and Chief People Officer, Seattle Children's

Seattle Children's has transformed Human Resources (HR), replacing its traditional HR structure and approaches with an integrated framework composed of teams dedicated to people and culture, talent acquisition, and workforce development. Aligned with the organization's Health Equity and Antiracism Action Plan and working closely with Seattle Children's Center for Diversity and

Health Equity, a large cross-functional team has been deployed to do the fundamental work of embedding equity and inclusion into the organization's culture and operations. Equity-focused initiatives have included tying executive compensation to specific equity, diversity, and inclusion dimensions (17% of pay is tied to achievement of equity-related goals); review and revision of more than 900 job descriptions; deployment of a variety of equity tools, including data equity dashboards to identify disparities by race, ethnicity, and language of care; building internal pathways toward leadership and management positions; de-emphasizing referrals as a key mechanism for sourcing new hires by removing the cash incentive; conducting a comprehensive evaluation of interview practices; leadership coaching; design of a robust onboarding process with ongoing engagement to support retention; and development of a diverse, representative hospital board of trustees. Seattle Children's has hired two recruiters who are focused on increasing the diversity of the applicant pool specifically for top leadership positions, according to Rosie Jones, Director of Talent Acquisition, with considerable success. Another effective strategy to diversify the applicant pool across various job types, as well as to further inclusion goals, has been to engage staff from Inclusion Networks (employee resource or affinity groups), with Inclusion Network leaders (who are compensated for their time and commitment to equity work) participating in interview panels during hiring, as well as in onboarding initiatives.

The organization's integrated People and Culture team emphasizes that the work of creating an inclusive workplace is about much more than recruitment and retention for open positions. Supporting values-based behavior is fundamental, with leaders committed to being proactive, accepting accountability, building trust and facilitating healing, and empowered to address challenges that might once have been "handed off" to HR staff. A forward-thinking approach to workforce development—cultivating talent—is equally important. "We're engaging earlier and earlier to build a diverse pipeline," says Wendy Price, Director of Workforce

Development Planning. Efforts to interest young people in the healthcare professions and in Seattle Children's have involved on-site, hands-on programs with middle, high school, and college students. Programs to engage young adults have included partnerships and sponsorships with community-based organizations and local workforce development initiatives.

An area of significant concern both nationally and for Seattle Children's is a shortage of nurses, and to address this challenge the hospital has developed an innovative nurse residency program for recent nursing graduates. The program prioritizes nurses who have a desire to work in an environment that "supports anti-racism and respects diversity and inclusiveness in an approach to individualized care." To increase the diversity of the applicant pool, the program has eliminated cash incentives for internal referrals and automatic interviews for all candidates referred internally, a strategy that has proven effective.

Messaging is an integral component of any change management effort, and the Seattle Children's People and Culture team advocates engaging a communications professional with expertise in antiracism and diversity, equity, and inclusion. Internal and external communications have focused on transparency and visibility (making people and culture and diversity, equity, and inclusion, and health equity data accessible), exposure and awareness, success stories, and sharing where progress is needed. Seattle Children's Hospital Board of Trustees has endorsed an integrated people and culture framework—values-based behavior, equity approaches to talent acquisition and workforce development, and antiracist communication practice—as a comprehensive business strategy, backed by substantial resources to help ensure success.

*Antiracism work is a journey. Our goal at Seattle Children's is for antiracist practices to be so deeply embedded in the way we operate, that we won't even realize it. Until we arrive at this place, the work will continue.*

Alicia Tieder, MSW, LICSW, MBA, Associate Vice President and Chief Health Equity Officer, Seattle Children's

## Recommended Reading and Resources

Byrd MY, Scott CL. *The Palgrave Handbook of Antiracism in Human Resource Development.* eBook. Palgrave Macmillan; 2024. https://doi.org/10.1007/978-3-031-52268-0

Daniels S. *The Anti-Racist Organization: Dismantling Systemic Racism in the Workplace.* Wiley & Sons; 2022.

National Minority Supplier Development Council. Accessed February 6, 2025. https://nmsdc.org

Winters MF and the Winters Group. *Racial Justice at Work: Practical Solutions for Systems Change.* Berrett–Koehler; 2023.

## References

1. Deloitte. 2024 Gen Z and Millennial Survey. Living and Working with Purpose in a Transforming World. 2024. https://www.deloitte.com/global/en/issues/work/content/genz-millennialsurvey.html?icid=gx:2or:3dp:4genzandmillennialsurvey2023:5GC1000102:6wok:20230517:deloitteinsights
2. Daniels S. *The Anti-Racist Organization: Dismantling Systemic Racism in the Workplace.* Wiley & Sons; 2022.
3. Minority Business Development Agency. Accessed February 6, 2025. https://www.mbda.gov/about/history
4. Health Research and Educational Trust. Increasing Supplier Diversity in Health Care. Chicago, IL. Health Research and Educational Trust. September 2015. https://www.hpoe.org
5. The National Minority Supplier Development Council. Accessed February 6, 2025. https://nmsdc.org
6. Seattle Children's. Health Equity and Antiracism Action Plan: Report Highlight: Workforce Diversity. Accessed February 10, 2025. https://www.seattlechildrens.org/about/commitment-anti-racism/report-highlight-workforce-diversity/

# 6
# Antiracist Leadership and Learning

Transforming policies and practices to prioritize health equity—from the collection of accurate sociodemographic patient data to the development of equitable supplier programs—is a complex, multifaceted undertaking. Learning and training opportunities for leaders and staff throughout the organization are an essential, yet often under-resourced, component of this large-scale effort. The intentional and active work to dismantle racism and sustain systemic change engages employees at all levels in approaching their roles in ways that may require new knowledge, skills, and behaviors. Nearly all organizational antiracism and health equity action plans or road maps include goals and objectives related to learning and training. Understanding the upstream drivers of structural racism and discrimination and their downstream impacts on health and well-being, the history of medical racism and health disparities, the ways in which racism operates in our organizations, and developing the skills to evolve inclusive workplace cultures and advance health equity are critically important.

In this chapter, we will consider antiracist leadership models and health equity–focused learning and training. Needs and resources for these fundamental components will vary considerably from organization to organization, as will the organizational infrastructure for training, which might include health equity centers, diversity councils or committees, human resources or career services, and talent development and learning offices. Many existing learning and training programs across the organization may be adaptable and scalable. Health equity and antiracism education and training curricula and toolkits are available from a variety of sources, as we will describe later in the chapter. Organizations with limited existing programs may want to investigate what peer organizations have implemented and found to be successful.

*Transforming Health Care*. Lynne D. Richardson and Sima Rabinowitz, Oxford University Press.
 DOI: 10.1093/oso/9780197805374.003.0007

## Implementing Learning and Training Plans

As they address institutional and structural policies that perpetuate racism, healthcare organizations must also strive to model and promote antiracist perspectives and behaviors. Eliminating racist practices and beliefs held by people in the organization is essential to meeting health equity goals.[1] Building or enhancing antiracist learning and practical skills development should begin, as should all of the initiatives we have described, with a review and assessment of the current context, including identification of learning and training needs for leadership and staff around antiracism and health equity; relevant education and training programs and materials that are already in place or can be modified or adapted, as well as an assessment of what may be missing; the groups and individuals who should be included in assessing, designing, and evaluating new learning and training programs and materials, including the engagement of community members; modes of program delivery (online learning and virtual platforms, e-learning options, on-site trainers and coaches, etc.); and the resources required to deploy antiracism learning and training opportunities throughout the organization. Conversations about racism and racial inequities can be difficult, and it may be useful to engage experienced facilitators to assist in leading antiracism training efforts.

It will be important to set specific goals and objectives for organization-wide learning and training, as well as for any department or role-specific training, which might include concentrated focus areas (bias reduction, cultural awareness, structural racism, understanding health disparities and social determinants of health, etc.) and requirements for participation (mandatory or elective programming based on role, setting, and goals), along with formal mechanisms to track progress (the percentage of staff who complete each training module annually by role and department or unit, etc.) and outcomes measures (for example, pre- and post-test assessment of the effectiveness of trainings, periodic pulse surveys) to determine how learning is put into practice and how organizational performance is impacted. As we have reiterated throughout this book, antiracism task forces, councils, and committees should involve the broad participation of leaders, staff, faculty, trainees/students, community leaders and advocates, and patients in their antiracism action plans, including in the development of approaches to learning and training. It may be useful to engage employee resource groups or affinity groups in helping to assess learning and training needs or in pilot testing materials.

Many organizations have created foundational or core learning curricula to support a common understanding of the basic terminology and concepts related to antiracism, health equity, and creating an inclusive workplace. At the same time, it is likely that some types of training will need to be designed expressly for specific groups of leaders or staff and tailored for different settings. A one-size-fits-all approach might seem most efficient in terms of time and resources but could be significantly less effective in helping everyone in the organization develop the understanding and skills needed to put what is learned into practice. Providing protected time on the job for participation in both mandatory and elective learning, and ensuring that staff at all levels are supported by their leaders and teams in engaging in antiracism and health equity learning and training, demonstrates the organization's commitment to becoming an equitable, antiracist healthcare organization and to equipping leaders and staff at all levels with the knowledge and skills to collaborate in this work.

## Modeling Antiracist Leadership

Senior leaders in every organization, regardless of its size, are responsible for establishing strategic priorities, setting goals, and allocating resources. Leaders convey their vision, aspirations, and expectations for the organization and help to shape workplace culture, not only through these decisions and choices but also through their actions and communications. Health and hospital system leaders committed to health equity should participate in antiracist learning, model antiracist behaviors, and actively support the development of a bias-free, inclusive environment for all staff and patients. Learning and training will be important to build the capacity of the organization's leaders to discuss race and racism and to develop awareness of the history and current impact of racism and discrimination in clinical, operational, and administrative settings, as well as to support them in leading the specific antiracism action plan initiatives for which they will be accountable.

A number of health and hospital systems across the country have opted to include their commitment to antiracism and health equity in recruitment materials and job descriptions for top leadership positions, tie compensation to achieving specific equity goals, and require engagement in antiracist leadership development or enrichment as a condition of employment. For these organizations, demonstrating or developing antiracist leadership skills is considered an essential leadership competency.

Antiracism leadership learning and training can take the form of on-site or virtual workshops and courses, small group activities, online learning programs, peer learning, or individual coaching and could include mandatory and elective options, depending on needs and resources. Antiracist leadership programs and curricula vary in approach, format, and content, but most incorporate several common goals and themes, which include, among others: (1) engaging in self-reflection and developing awareness of how our own racial and ethnic identity and life experiences influence our daily decisions and behaviors; (2) understanding the history of structural racism and medical racism and the institution's role in this history; (3) learning to recognize bias and identify discriminatory policies and practices throughout the organization; (4) cultivating the skills to lead others in difficult conversations about race and racism, build trust, and promote an inclusive workplace; and (5) gaining deep cultural awareness, including a nuanced understanding of cultural differences and diverse perspectives.

Many organizational change management and systems change leadership models include concepts that are relevant and important for antiracist leadership, specifically the capacity to bring people together around a shared vision, to drive both adaptive change (addressing complex challenges) and technical change (addressing contained or more narrowly defined problems with specific solutions), and to mentor and develop others. The goal to develop others and to engage in succession planning is critical. The work to become an antiracist organization focused on achieving health equity cannot depend only on the vision or effort of current leadership but must be sustainable as changes in leadership occur.

Antiracist leadership models in health care are relatively new. There are no accepted standards, nor is there any consensus around what types of training or learning content may be most effective. Most antiracism and health equity action plans include cultivating antiracist leadership practices among the organizational strategies to be implemented and evaluated, even if they do not describe plans for formal leadership models. Strategies from bias-reduction training, such as the inclusion of case studies and scenarios, using real-world examples, role play, simulation, and perspective-taking (imagining the experiences of others) may be particularly effective.[2–4] Leaders who participate in ongoing learning will demonstrate a commitment to professional and personal growth and to creating and sustaining a learning organization. Curricula might include specific themes related to action plan or road map initiatives, training tailored to meet the needs specifically of individuals who are new to leadership, and courses or workshops customized to meet needs as they arise through implementation of the action plan or as suggested by leaders in post-training evaluation and other forms of feedback.

## Learning and Training to Support Individual and Organizational Development

Many health system and community leaders share the belief that it is necessary to tackle the issue of racism in health care and train the healthcare workforce around issues of racial inequities to achieve health equity.[1,5] Across the various offices or departments that are responsible for organization-wide training, learning and training programs and resources could encompass both general themes and practices (implicit bias, allyship) and specific content and skills associated with action plan or road map strategies. Although they may be related, developing a general understanding of how to recognize and manage one's own biases is distinct from learning how to tell patients about why collecting their race, ethnicity, and preferred language data is important and how to do so in a respectful, culturally responsive manner. And while all staff should gain a basic understanding of the social determinants of health, training on how to screen for them will be role and setting specific.

In many ways, learning around antiracism and health equity is not significantly different from other types of training that support the enhancement of knowledge and development of skills and competencies to improve individual performance and contribute to the organization's effectiveness and success. Nonetheless, few subjects in American life and institutions may be as challenging and fraught with tension as race and racism. Approaches to training around antiracism and bias reduction, therefore, invariably describe creating a safe environment for engaging in courageous conversations while employing strategies that encourage people to expect, and accept, a certain degree of discomfort. Training of any type (online courses, virtual workshops, small or large group meetings) for people in any role (clinicians, allied health professionals, operations teams, administrative staff) with clear applicability to people's day-to-day work, and which supports the development of practical skills, is likely to be the most welcomed and effective. When new training curricula or programs are being developed or considered for organization-wide implementation, it may be useful to pilot them first in one or two departments or units, collect feedback from participants, and refine and improve them before rolling them out to the larger organization.

Evidence from hundreds of antiracism and diversity, equity, and inclusion trainings across multiple areas of practice, settings, and roles suggests that among the most successful strategies are a longitudinal training design (as opposed to one-time trainings), targeted skill building, prioritizing both individual and organizational development and change, and the use of validated instruments for evaluation.[6] We will focus briefly here on a few of the most prevalent learning and training themes for the healthcare workforce around dismantling racism in health care.

## Antibias Training

Antibias or bias reduction interventions are not new, of course. Unconscious bias training has been common in business and academic settings for decades, with more recent adoption in health and hospital systems. There is considerable disagreement about the effectiveness of these programs, which vary significantly in approach and quality. It is widely understood that simply making people aware of stereotypes and prejudice is not sufficient to prevent or reduce bias or discrimination and that one-and-done approaches are inadequate to help people disrupt lifelong habits and develop new ways of thinking or behaving. However, antibias and bias-reduction training (implicit bias, microaggressions, allyship) may be most effective when it employs approaches that bring people together to support collaboration and partnerships across identity lines and engage participants in recognizing specific challenges and designing solutions. Trainings should address specific clinical issues related to communities served by the organization, present real-world scenarios and experiential learning that simulate real-life interactions and communication, and offer opportunities for deep understanding of the perspectives of others.[4,7,8]

### Implicit Bias

The terms implicit bias and unconscious bias are often used interchangeably. We will use the term implicit bias here to describe attitudes that may underlie or affect our actions and decisions based on unconscious or involuntary favoring or disfavoring of an individual or group. These behaviors may arise from stereotypes, prejudice, misperceptions, misinformation, or other sources that drive us to act in ways that can unfairly advantage or disadvantage an individual or group. Understanding and addressing implicit bias in health care may be especially important, because although people in the health professions actively seek to do good and avoid intentionally causing harm, we know that bias and discrimination continue to influence care and can have a profoundly adverse impact on patient outcomes.

Addressing implicit bias as a means to reducing inequities in care and disparities in outcomes is understood by many to be essential. As of the writing of this book, seven states had mandated implicit bias training for some healthcare providers (California, Delaware, Maryland, Michigan, Minnesota, New Jersey, and Washington state), often as a component of larger equity training efforts, and all of these states require implicit bias training for maternal health providers. California's mandatory Dignity in Pregnancy and Childbirth Project, which includes implicit bias training, was designed for both clinicians and hospital management in response to the state's Dignity in Pregnancy and Childbirth legislation.[9] At least two dozen additional states have similar legislation pending.[10–13] In Washington state, mandated health equity training for all health professionals (doctors, nurses, dentists, pharmacists, chiropractors, mental health professionals), with regular renewal of state credentialing, must include implicit bias training, among other themes.[14,15]

Although there are no standardized national training curricula for implicit bias training, experts agree that training based on real cases, created with input from clinicians, staff, and—above all—the input of patients, is more effective than training based on hypothetical scenarios or static online programming that lacks interactive components. The goal is to help participants develop empathy and an awareness of biases and what gives rise to them and have the capacity both to understand and to imagine others' experiences and points of view. For this reason, even self-administered online training should include opportunities for self-reflection and introspection.

## Microaggressions

The term microaggressions is often used to refer to subtle acts, verbal or nonverbal, that reinforce stereotypes and discriminatory social norms around identity (race, ethnicity, gender, sexuality, disability). When the term was first defined more than a half century ago, it was used specifically in the context of anti-Black racism to highlight the cumulative negative effect these subtle offenses have on Black people.[16] Interest in microaggressions as an important social phenomenon, including in healthcare organizations, has recently surged, with a 770% increase in research papers on racial microaggressions from 2000 to 2024.[17,18]

Racial microaggressions may take a number of forms and cause distinct types of harm. Examples commonly found in training curricula include assumptions about background, training, and competence; remarks about appearance; persistent interruption of Black colleagues when they are speaking or dismissing their remarks altogether; excluding Black colleagues or team members from group activities or plans; mistaking Black coworkers for one another (misidentifying); addressing everyone in the room by their title or an honorific with the exception of Black colleagues; and tokenism (including a single Black member in a larger group that is intended to be diverse), among others. Individual-level microaggressions can be compounded by organizational-level offenses, which could include the absence of Black people in images and artwork in materials used or posted throughout the hospital, for example, or naming a building or facility for someone who is known to hold or have held racist views and attitudes.

The "micro" in microaggression does not mean that these offenses are inconsequential or that their impact is small. The harm they inflict can be deep and lasting. Micro refers instead to the fact that these forms of aggression may seem invisible to everyone except those whom they target. Although more explicit and overt forms of racism and discrimination are not socially acceptable in most settings, microaggressions often go unnoticed and unaddressed, and they may be no less damaging. One goal of training around microaggressions is, in fact, to make them visible.

It is imperative to ensure that everyone in the organization can work in an environment that is free of bias and discrimination. Healthcare organizations have developed trainings to address microaggressions among coworkers, as well as among providers and patients. Training to address microaggressions often includes helping participants understand the many forms microaggressions can take and the ways in which they inflict harm; developing the skills to recognize verbal and nonverbal microaggressions, along with strategies for disarming them (ways to let others know when a microaggression has been committed and to initiate a dialogue to address it);

and practicing the skills and techniques to address microaggressions as they occur. Underlying all learning and training around microaggressions is the fundamental understanding that it is not the responsibility of those who are the target of microaggressions to interrupt them or teach others about them in the moment or attempt to address them after the fact. For this reason, many trainings on microaggressions include discussion of allyship and emphasize the need to focus on building concrete skills to address microaggressions.

## Allyship

Many healthcare systems require employees to participate in bystander training, the development of techniques for an observer or witness to support someone who may be harmed or is at risk of harm by diffusing or de-escalating a potentially hostile, abusive, or dangerous situation. Allyship, instead, is direct intervention by a member of a dominant group who seeks to actively change practices, policies, or even the culture of an organization that serve, however unintentionally, to marginalize or oppress minoritized groups. An ally, on witnessing a microaggression (for example, a Black female colleague is interrupted every time she begins to speak), might ask a question or make a remark to raise awareness or directly address the bias underlying an action (*"I think you may not realize that you have interrupted Dr. X every time she has tried to contribute to our conversation."*) Perhaps one of the most important aspects of allyship is acting in the moment to address immediate issues, rather than later commiserating with a colleague who has been harmed or mentioning the incident as a side remark in a later meeting. Allyship is not about confrontation, but instead about attempting to intervene on attitudes and behaviors, speaking up for others, and making it safe to challenge or disrupt the status quo on behalf of others.

As a form of bias reduction, training around allyship is often incorporated into implicit or unconscious bias training or included with learning around microaggressions. Similar to other types of bias-reduction training, programs built around real-world scenarios and opportunities to develop and practice concrete techniques and practical skills may be most effective, especially given that allyship is about the capacity for, and willingness to engage in, formulating an active response. Allyship can allow those who believe in racial equity to put their beliefs into practice, something that many people working in the health professions wish to do.[3,19]

### Responding to Explicit Bias or Discriminatory Behavior

As we described in Chapter 5, many healthcare organizations have developed codes of conduct for patients, families, and visitors clearly stating that racist speech and behaviors are unacceptable. Aligned with these formal policies, organizations may also offer training in strategies for responding to explicit bias or discriminatory behavior, with guidance and practical skills for specific settings, such as the emergency department or inpatient care. Trainings could include approaches to support a zero-tolerance culture for explicitly racist speech or behavior in the workplace and information about when and how to engage managers, supervisors, or other leaders in addressing specific instances of overt racial hostility or discrimination observed or experienced by anyone in the organization. Although some general training programs may be broadly beneficial, training tailored to specific roles might have the greatest impact, particularly if the goal is to have a direct impact on patient care.

## Training in Health Disparities/Health Equity

Healthcare organizations that have established health equity as a strategic priority should incorporate discussion of health equity themes in onboarding activities and materials for leaders and staff throughout the organization and include health equity themes in regular organizational communications. The equity measures and data from disparities dashboards described in Chapter 2 can serve as the basis for the development of health equity learning and training for presentations, workshops, or training curricula and other resources (fact sheets, toolkits, etc.) that can be tailored for specific departments, units, and/or roles and focus on specific priority populations.

Health disparities and health equity learning can also happen more informally, through the intentional application of an equity lens to plans and communications that may not necessarily be centered on equity themes. New practices or policies, or changes to existing ones, that will impact all patients either directly or indirectly, for example, should reflect consideration of which patients might be advantaged or disadvantaged. Mechanisms for soliciting input or feedback on programs or initiatives that are not focused on equity/disparities could include questions about how equity concerns might be addressed to improve or refine these initiatives.

## Antiracism and Health Equity Learning and Training Resources for Health and Hospital Systems

Health equity and antiracism learning and training curricula, tools, and other resources are available from many sources. Healthcare leaders seeking guidance and existing resources might begin with national and local governmental agencies such as the Centers for Disease Control and Prevention, the Department of Health and Human Services, the Centers for Medicare & Medicaid Services, and state, county, or city public health departments and offices. Nearly every state has established infrastructure to address health equity, and many post links to educational materials and training resources and opportunities.[10] Some state, city, and large regional training centers offer health equity and related resources and training opportunities through divisions and offices of public health. Many academic medical centers across the country publish lists of antiracism and health equity resources on public-facing library or educational program websites, often with links to health equity toolkits and training tools.

Professional societies and associations across numerous disciplines and health professions also post information about antiracism or health equity resources on their websites, including education and training toolkits, and information about training programs, continuing education opportunities, and certificate programs. Community-based organizations may also be able to provide guidance, as well as links to training resources around relevant health equity and racial health justice themes, and/or offer learning opportunities. Local, regional, and national nonprofit organizations, as well as consulting firms led by experienced professionals and practitioners, offer a range of services, from learning needs assessment to the design and delivery of customized training programs, including antiracist and health equity–focused leadership development.

## Antiracism in Schools of Medicine, Nursing, and the Health Sciences

Since about 2010, educators in most medical, nursing, public health, and health sciences schools and programs (social work, occupational health, physical therapy, nutrition and dietetics) have revised curricula to incorporate knowledge and skills related to health disparities and inequities, often in response to guidance from professional associations and accreditation bodies.[21] More recently, although to a lesser extent, many schools have incorporated curricula or clinical training components focused more specifically on antiracism. These efforts range from large-scale curricular transformation at a few institutions, to the integration of new content into existing courses, to the addition of optional educational modules or training opportunities. Relatively few medical education programs have robust antiracism curricula, however.[22] Some schools have engaged in more comprehensive or holistic efforts to advance antiracism and equity throughout their institutions with initiatives to implement antiracist, equitable policies and practices beyond the curriculum to include admissions, student affairs, and their own governance structures, among other functions.

Learning collaboratives—discipline-specific institutions or programs (medical education, nursing, family medicine) that come together to consider best practices, co-create curricula or training, and develop evaluation metrics and processes—seek both to dismantle racism and advance health equity at their own institutions and to inform and influence education and training on a national level. As we briefly described in the introduction to this book, as the national landscape evolves, it is difficult to predict how new federal and/or state policies and regulations may impact education and training in medicine, nursing, and the health sciences. A learning collaborative approach may be particularly useful going forward to help ensure that antiracist, health equity–focused education and training can be part of a larger national agenda. Working collaboratively, organizations can support each other in interpreting and addressing regulatory and legislative changes, developing training for faculty and staff, and engaging in advocacy.

## Developing Understanding and Skills for Antiracist Practice

Achieving health equity will require a clinical workforce with both an understanding of the structural and systemic factors that perpetuate racial health disparities and the specific skills and competency to engage in antiracist practice. Many of the strategies and best practices for antiracism and health equity–focused training for health and hospital system leaders and employees described throughout this chapter are also applicable for medical, nursing, and health sciences education. These include communicating a unifying terminology (ensuring that everyone has a common understanding of key terms and themes); engaging experienced teachers, trainers, and facilitators with specific expertise in antiracism learning and training to lead courses and workshops; using case studies, real-world scenarios, and inclusive role play and simulation strategies; providing specific action steps and concrete tools; and engaging communities, as relevant, in the design and delivery of population-focused training.

Academic institutions with multiple schools, a medical school, a college of pharmacy, and a school of nursing, for example, or with multiple health sciences programs, might consider developing interprofessional learning opportunities to promote a shared understanding of, and commitment to, antiracist practice across disciplines. This could be useful in helping to amplify antiracist approaches across disciplines as they translate to practice and, perhaps, to close the gap that can exist between academic training and the culture of hospital systems.

## Learning and Training for Transformation

The work to dismantle racism and achieve racial equity is a long journey that will continue to evolve. Disrupting decades of bias and discrimination is urgent, but will take time. Organizations aiming to embed system-wide antiracist principles, practices, and policies will want to align training and learning with the goal of large-scale transformation. Engaging everyone in the organization in ongoing learning and training underscores the seriousness and complexity of this work and can allow for continuous change and improvement.

## Summary

1. Incorporate health equity learning and antiracist skills development into organizational action plans or road maps with learning and training opportunities for leaders and staff at all levels.
2. Assess current leadership and training programs, identify opportunities to adapt or build on these resources, and include leaders and staff, as well as community members and patients, in the design and evaluation of new training curricula and tools.
3. Include general themes such as implicit bias and microaggressions, and specific training around action plan or road map goals in training for leaders and staff.
4. Promote understanding of the need to reduce racial bias and discrimination as integral to the goal of achieving health equity.
5. Consider the development of an antiracist leadership model detailing the priorities, principles, and practices expected of antiracist leaders and develop training to support best practices.
6. Incorporate real-world scenarios, development of practical skills, and the clear applicability of training to day-to-day work and accountabilities in antiracism learning and training. Tailor training to specific settings or roles, as needed and relevant.
7. Implement longitudinal, ongoing training, where possible; this is likely to be more successful than one-time training approaches and will demonstrate a commitment to racial equity as a priority and reinforce the importance of continuous learning and improvement.

**SPOTLIGHT**

## A Learning Collaborative Grounded in Systems Change

*In order to understand how to address structural racism, we have to understand the parts, the relationships, and the interactions that contribute to it as a whole.*

Ann Gakumo, PhD, RN, Associate Dean for Inclusion and Community Impact; Co-Director, Structural Racism in Nursing Academia project; University of Cincinnati College of Nursing

Structural Racism in Nursing Academia, a national initiative to advance antiracism in nursing education led by the University of Cincinnati College of Nursing, is grounded in the understanding that systems change will require a collaborative effort. With the support of a grant from the Josiah Macy Foundation, the College's equity leaders have convened a Learning Collaborative of 13 institutions from throughout the United States with the goal of creating evidence-based programs to dismantle structural racism in nursing education and promote antiracist practices and policies. Collaborating institutions participated in the American Association of Colleges of Nursing Leading Across Multidimensional Perspectives Climate and Culture Survey (LAMP), which assesses the experiences of students, faculty, and staff at nursing schools to identify practices that facilitate student and professional success and a sense of belonging, along with the characteristics that facilitate engagement and can drive institutional decision-making and meaningful change.

The Collaborative includes both public and private schools of nursing with on-site, hybrid, and online curricula committed to developing antiracist programs across five key areas: (1) curriculum and pedagogy, (2) inclusion and belonging for students, (3) inclusion and belonging for faculty, (4) academic culture and environment, and (5) clinical environment. The Collaborative's work is informed by theoretical concepts, specifically intergroup conflict theory and transformational systems change. The group meets monthly on a virtual platform and is joined by an advisory board of national leaders in nursing and guest presenters who offer practical guidance and share their expertise.

The project is ambitious: Participating schools must develop programs and evaluation plans for all five areas to be completed during the three-year grant period. Greer Glazer, Dean Emeritus of the College of Nursing and Co-Director of the Structural Racism in Nursing Academia project, emphasizes that while the work is challenging and time-consuming, the purpose of the Collaborative is to enable schools to learn from each other to support and accelerate the process of evolving, implementing, and evaluating their antiracist nursing education programs.

Institutional leadership, dedicated resources, good data from an inclusive group of stakeholders, and the agility to pivot in the context of a changing national landscape are critical, the project team explains, and it is important to think about engaging with partners beyond schools of nursing, both more broadly across the institution and in the local community. The Cincinnati team cautions that identifying problems and solutions is just one part of the work; transforming systems often involves rethinking and revising bylaws and policies and understanding every change as part of a larger transformational effort.

The opportunity to collaborate has been one of the most impactful aspects of the project, according to Sean Brown, RN, a graduate of the University of Cincinnati's College of Nursing and the Learning Collaborative's Senior Project Manager. Following a successful in-person retreat, participants have requested annual retreats, saying that working together has helped them address some of the barriers they have encountered, both within and beyond their institutions. The Learning Collaborative is facilitating implementation of antiracism programs at the individual institutions, with the goal of broader replication at schools of nursing across the country, says Project Manager Jordan Gayle. Project leaders Ann Gakumo and Glazer have found that a great deal of important and innovative work to dismantle racism in nursing education is underway around the country, but too little of this work has been shared. They hope that Learning Collaborative schools will lead the way in disseminating this work where colleagues in nursing and leaders across the spectrum of healthcare settings will have access to it.

> *It doesn't matter if you're new to antiracism work, you can still do this, and it has to be done. Everyone can be a leader.*
> Greer Glazer, PhD, RN, CNP, FANN, Dean Emeritus and Schmidlapp Professor of Nursing; University of Cincinnati College of Nursing

## Recommended Reading and Resources

America's Essential Hospitals. Currently Engaging Topics: Structural Racism. Accessed February 6, 2025. https://essentialhospitals.org/?s=structural+racism&fwp=1

American Medical Association. Health Equity Education Center. Accessed February 6, 2025. https://edhub.ama-assn.org/health-equity-ed-center

American Association of Colleges of Medicine. MedEdPORTAL. Anti-racism Collection. Accessed March 21, 2025. https://www.medportal.org/anti-racism

Artiga S, Rao A. State reported efforts to address health disparities: A 50-state review. Kaiser Family Foundation. November 22, 2024. https://www.kff.org/racial-equity-and-health-policy/issue-brief/state-reported-efforts-to-address-health-disparities-a-50-state-review/

Association of American Family Physicians. EveryOne Toolkit. Implicit Bias Resources. Accessed February 6, 2025. https://www.aafp.org/family-physician/patient-care/the-everyone-project/toolkit/implicit-bias.html

Institute for Healthcare Improvement. Accessed February 6, 2025. https://www.ihi.org/improvement-areas/improvement-area-health-equity

Novack DH, Burnett C. Antiracism in Health Care Curriculum Guide. Drexel University Center for Professionalism and Communication in Health Care. Accessed March 23, 2025. https://webcampus.med.drexel.edu/pchc/

Rural Health Information Hub. Rural Health Equity Toolkit. School of Medicine and Sciences. Grand Fork, North Dakota. Accessed February 6, 2025. https://www.ruralhealthinfo.org/toolkits/health-equity

## References

1. Weissman JS, Adler RR, Betancour J, Tan-Mcgory A, Lewis JA, DesRoches CM. How hospitals are addressing the effects of racism: A mixed-methods study of hospital equity officers. *Health Aff.* 2023; 42(10): 1402–1410. https://doi.org/10.1377/hlthaff.2023.00474

2. Fricke M, Ducharne DB, Beavis A, Flett P, Ossman S. Addressing racism in the workplace through simulation: So much to unlearn. *Frontiers Rehabil Sci.* March 30, 2023. https://doi.org/10.3389/fresc.2023.1126085
3. Ayub N, Regalia C, Wilson T, Gaught C, Anderson C, Banerjee D. Theater for Health Care Equity: A model for inclusion and anti-bias training in academic medicine. *R I MedJ*2024 June: 29–34. http://rimed.org/rimedicaljournal/2024/06/2024-06-29-contribution-ayub.pdf
4. Schmader T, Dennehey TC, Baron AC. Why antibias interventions (need not) fail. *Perspect Psychol Sci.* 2022; 1–23. https://doi.org/10.1177/17456916211057565
5. Robert Wood Johnson Foundation. Justice Squared. Just Leaders for a Just Health System. Program Design. 2024. https://justicesquared.org/wp-content/uploads/2024/10/Justice-Squared-Program-Design-FINAL-10.21.24-.pdf
6. Wang ML, Gomes A, Rosa M, Copeland P, Santana VJ. A systematic review of diversity, equity, and inclusion and antiracism training studies: Findings and future directions. *Transl Behav Med.* 2024; 14:156–171. https://doi.org/10.1093/tbm/ibad061
7. Cooper L, Saha S, van Ryn M. Mandated implicit bias training for health professionals—a step toward equity in health care. *JAMA Health Forum.* 2022; 3(8):e223250. 10.1001/jamahealthforum.2022.3250
8. Garrett SB, Jones L, Montague A, Fa-Yusuf H, Harris-Taylor J, Powell B, et al. Challenges and opportunities for clinician implicit bias training: Insights from perinatal care stakeholders. *HEQ.* 2023; 7(1):506–519. https://doi.org/10.1089/heq.2023.0126
9. Humanitas Institute. Meeting Multifaceted Needs: A Guide for Perinatal Care Providers. Accessed February 18, 2025. https://www.humanitasinst.org/ca-ab-2319
10. Artiga S, Rao A. State reported efforts to address health disparities: A 50-state review. Kaiser Family Foundation. November 22, 2024. https://www.kff.org/racial-equity-and-health-policy/issue-brief/state-reported-efforts-to-address-health-disparities-a-50-state-review/
11. Montague A, Hooper S. *Introduced Implicit Bias Training Bills in the United States, 2019–2022. Multi-Stakeholder Engagement with State Policies to Advance Antiracism in Maternal Health (MEND) Study Reporting.* University of California, San Francisco; 2023. https://pretermbirthca.ucsf.edu/sites/g/files/tkssra2851/f/Introduced%20IBT%20Bills%20Chart_v03.1.pdf
12. Garrett SB, Jones L, Montague A, Fa-Yusuf H, Harris-Taylor J, Powell B, et al. Challenges and opportunities for clinician implicit bias training: Insights from perinatal care stakeholders. *HEQ.* 2023; 7(1):506–519. https://doi.org/10.1089/heq.2023.0126
13. University of California, San Francisco. California Pre-term Birth Initiative. Accessed February 6, 2025. https://pretermbirthca.ucsf.edu/currently-funded-projects/multi-stakeholder-engagement-state-policies-advance-antiracism-maternal
14. CE Group Washington Health Equity CE Course. Accessed February 6, 2025. https://washington-health-equity-ce.com

15. Washington State Board of Nursing. New Health Equity Continuing Education Requirements. Accessed February 18, 2025. https://nursing.wa.gov/licensing/maintain-license/continuing-competency
16. Pierce C. Offensive mechanisms. In: Barbour F, ed. *The Black Seventies.* Porter Sargent; 1970.
17. Osman M, Williams MT, Alftieh A. State of the science of racial microaggressions. *Behav Ther.* 2024; 55:1172–1188. https://doi.org/10.1016/j.beth.2024.05.005
18. Freeman L, Stewart H. *Microaggressions in Medicine.* Oxford University Press; 2024.
19. Wu D, Lamercie S-H, Pineda H, Hessler D, Saba G, Salazar R, et al. The efficacy of an anti-oppression curriculum for health professionals. *Fam Med.* 2019; 10(30):21–29. https://journals.stfm.org/familymedicine/2019/january/wu-2018-0079/
20. Shani SR, Gonzalez CM, Zhang C, Hassan I. Structural competency: A faculty development workshop series for anti-racism in medical education. *MedEdPORTAL.* 2025; 21:11492. https://doi.org/10.15766/mep_2374-8265.11492
21. Falusi O, Chun-Seeley L, de la Torre D, Dooley DG, Baiyewu M, Gborkorquellie TT, Merrill CT, et al. Teaching the teachers: Development and evaluation of a racial health equity curriculum for faculty. *MedEdPORTAL.* 2023; 19:11305. https://doi.org/10.15766/mep_2374-8265.11305
22. Fatahi G, Racic M, Rocher-Miranda MI, Patterson DG, Phelan S, et al. The current state of antiracism curricula in undergraduate and graduate medical education: A qualitative study of US academic health centers. *Ann Fam Med.* 2023; 21:S14–S21. https://doi.org/10.1370/afm.2919

# 7

# Multisector Partnerships

## Creating and Sustaining Change

Racial disparities in health resulting from the social and economic drivers of health are due, in large measure, to disinvestment, underinvestment, and neglect over many decades in communities across the country—both urban and rural. The existence of these conditions is a societal failure that neither government action nor market forces have corrected. Multisector initiatives to help improve the physical environment and/or the economic strength of local communities can have enormous impacts on health in that community. Healthcare organizations and systems have an important role to play in turning societal disinvestment and inattention into engagement, investment, and opportunities to thrive. In this chapter, we will consider strategies for working across sectors and industries to help solve problems and improve the lives and health of individuals and families in our communities. This can be accomplished by working collectively to foster inclusive and equitable local economies, engage communities effectively as partners, innovate effective and equitable business and payor models, and advocate for policy change. Although the systems and structures within which we work can seem too complex or deeply entrenched to change, with intention, effort, innovation, and commitment, they can be transformed to deliver more equitable health outcomes.

### Investing in Communities: The Anchor Mission

Health and hospital systems are fundamental economic assets in communities across the country.[1] As large mission-driven employers,

*Transforming Health Care*. Lynne D. Richardson and Sima Rabinowitz, Oxford University Press.
 DOI: 10.1093/oso/9780197805374.003.0008

hospitals, together with universities, have for many decades been characterized as anchor institutions, in other words, organizations that essentially anchor local economies through direct and indirect impacts. Anchor institutions account for a significant proportion of regional employment (9% on average), income (6.3% on average), and gross value added (the value of goods and services produced in a specific region minus the cost of the intermediate inputs used to create those goods and services: 8.1% on average), with a huge increase in all of these factors nationwide since the early 2000s.[2]

Many healthcare organizations and hospital systems have embraced their anchor role and are advancing an anchor mission, serving as either a convening or a core member of local multisector collectives and networks composed of other local or regional organizations. The anchor concept provides an excellent model for working collectively and collaboratively across sectors to address the structural drivers of health and contribute to creating inclusive, equitable local economies. This approach provides an opportunity to operationalize antiracist and health equity–focused perspectives and practices beyond single organizations, reinforcing their primacy internally while extending their reach and impact. Finally, during times when the political landscape is uncertain or may present new challenges, robust multisector collaboratives can persist together in their work and address these challenges with collective strength and ingenuity.

## Multisector Collaboratives

Many aspects of the anchor approach can be useful for health and hospital systems wishing to establish or expand multisector partnerships, even if establishing a formal anchor collaborative is not viable or of interest. Like many collectives and networks, healthcare anchor collaboratives often evolve from more narrowly focused local initiatives with a small group of partners and expand to include new partners and additional goals or shift focus in response to an emerging crisis such as the COVID-19 pandemic or an extreme local weather event.

The core composition of anchor collaboratives across the country varies significantly and may include multiple hospitals, health systems, other types of healthcare organizations, colleges and universities, community colleges and technical or business schools, city and county agencies, financial institutions, large corporations and corporate foundations, community-based organizations, faith-based organizations, community development agencies, public school systems, public libraries, and arts and cultural organizations, with all of these organizations engaging their own networks of additional neighborhood or community groups through work groups, committees, advisory boards, and project-based teams. An advantage of participating in broad multisector networks, and a valuable aspect of the anchor mission approach, is the opportunity to engage with new partners, especially those from sectors that, on the surface, may appear to be unrelated to health care.

The Healthcare Anchor Network (HAN), a national network of more than 75 health and hospital systems and allied organizations launched in 2017, has developed outstanding freely available resources, including detailed playbooks, to support organizations in developing effective anchor collaboratives.[3] The Anchor Institutions Task Force (AITF), a national think tank and movement of more than 1,000 individual members established in 2009, offers resources and opportunities to learn about and extend democratic cross-sector engagement in neighborhoods, cities, and regions to meet the needs of communities.[4] As we have reiterated throughout this book, a best practice in planning large equity-focused initiatives is to begin with an assessment of the current organizational context, in this case, identifying and connecting with existing multisector partnerships and community engagement efforts and activities throughout the organization.

### Shared Purpose and Principles

The individual organizations engaged in multisector partnerships and networks have different missions, organizational structures, processes and policies, perspectives, approaches to framing and solving problems, data needs and capacity, financial resources, ways of communicating, and levels of engagement with communities and with antiracist and equity-focused practices. To be effective, the participating organizations should articulate a clear shared purpose or imperative. Anchor healthcare collaboratives have, for example, elected to focus on objectives related to particular health conditions such as cancer or chronic illness; specific overarching health goals, such as life expectancy; or specific populations, such as maternal health or adolescent health or, in many cases, combinations of these. Clarity about, and commitment to, a shared purpose serves to unify partners' efforts and should inform internal and external communications and outreach about the collaborative's work.

The core principles driving the anchor collaborative movement are important for any type or size of multisector partnership focused on equity: building trusted relationships; engaging the communities most impacted; shifting power to ensure equitable decision-making; and supporting authentic dialogue and honest, transparent, and open communication, as well as the desire and will to learn from and with each other. Many anchor collaboratives formalize learning and outreach by hosting information sessions or events featuring community leaders and experts, and other types of public programs, along with educational activities intended specifically for collaborative member organizations.

## Frameworks and Infrastructure

The Healthcare Anchor Network structures goals for local impact around three broad strategies for inclusive economic growth and community wealth building: workforce, purchasing, and place-based investing. Regardless of the areas of focus targeted for impact or the specific initiatives undertaken, to be effective, multisector collaboratives will want to formalize the operational components of their collective work. It is essential to identify and secure the staff and resources to serve as strategic or backbone support (much like the strategies we described in Chapter 1) to oversee coordination and management of the collaboratives' activities and communications and to develop processes for equitable decision-making, which must include the engagement of those in the community who have been harmed by decades of disadvantage. It is critical to have robust data on local socioeconomic factors and conditions to inform decisions about how and where to focus the collaborative's efforts and to support the setting of goals. Once specific areas of focus have been identified and measurable time-bound targets and benchmarks have been established, collaboratives should select an evaluation framework and create a process for assessing progress toward short- and long-term impacts. Evaluation is an area where engaging expert consultants may be particularly useful or necessary.

Building robust and effective multisector collaboratives requires strong leadership buy-in and engagement and a substantial commitment of time. Our "Suggested Reading and Resources" at the conclusion of the chapter include a number of excellent tools to support healthcare organizations or hospital systems in standing up, engaging in, and sustaining effective anchor collaboratives.

## The Business Case and Impact Strategies

Multisector collaboratives and networks established to create and sustain well-being economies[5] are not charitable organizations. While many health and hospital systems participate in community giving, advancing the anchor mission is not a form of philanthropy, but instead a commitment to leveraging each participating organization's economic assets and resources in partnership with local communities for mutual benefit.[3] Anchor strategies and goals are designed to address specific organizational priorities while contributing to communities that have experienced economic disinvestment and disadvantage.

The Healthcare Anchor Network's core impact strategies—workforce, purchasing, investing—provide a useful way to organize approaches to fuel economic growth and community wealth building. We will briefly summarize a few of the many types of initiatives in which anchor collaboratives are engaging across the country, in partnership with, and guided by, local communities to address the needs and interests they have identified.

### Workforce

Access to thriving-wage jobs is a critical issue in communities across the country. Anchor collaboratives have developed effective strategies to address the workforce needs of their partner organizations while contributing to greater local economic well-being. In collaboration with local community-based organizations (CBOs) and neighborhood associations, healthcare organizations have established recruitment hubs focused on targeted hiring from specific neighborhoods or regions, as well as on-the-job training and career advancement initiatives designed around high-need positions within their organizations. Recruitment hubs can support low-income communities by providing access to computer stations and Internet services for job seekers, information and counseling related to local educational and training opportunities, and related types of information and assistance.

Organizations work with their Human Resources and talent acquisition teams to support anchor workforce initiatives, including setting target goals, revising or designing hiring policies to promote inclusive and equitable practices, developing toolkits to guide implementation of new programs and outreach, and educating and training staff throughout the organization to help meet anchor workforce recruitment goals. By collaborating with local colleges and vocational schools, job placement agencies, and CBOs, hospitals can help support employees who are hired through these initiatives with job coaching and mentoring, tuition support for ongoing education or training, and links to needed wraparound services, such as child care or transit vouchers, among other supports.

Anchor collaborative job opportunity and recruitment dashboards, with aggregated data across member organizations, can help identify gaps and needs and can track and monitor progress toward meeting goals. Health systems may want to explore opportunities to integrate workforce and place-based investment strategies, for example, through the development of job recruitment or training hubs located within multiuse facilities supported by anchor collaborative investment.

### Local Purchasing

Anchor collaborative impact purchasing initiatives are very much like the health system supplier diversity programs described in Chapter 5. They involve targeted efforts to source and purchase supplies and services from local businesses, including minority-owned, women-owned, or disabled-owned businesses, and to empower these groups through capacity-building programs and partnerships, such as coaching, advising, and mentoring. Collaboratives typically set both collaborative-wide and organizational targets for percentage of spend and/or number of local firms engaged. Many anchor collaboratives leverage their pooled assets to support local businesses through small grant awards or incubator programs to help grow start-ups. Purchasing can range from limited support, for example, contracting with a minority-owned local caterer for an on-site event, to major contracts for hospital supplies or the purchase of locally grown produce for hospital food service units.

Collaborating across sectors can generate powerful opportunities for local businesses to grow and thrive while benefiting each organization's priorities and business goals, including jointly contracting for various services (for example, administrative support services or laundry and linen services). Anchor collaborative members can partner to create a database of local vendors and suppliers, along with dashboards to track progress, and might consider jointly offering programs to promote impact purchasing throughout their own organizations and in the community.

### Place-Based Investing

Socially responsible investing, also known as impact investing, is not new. In the context of the anchor collaboratives described here, place-based investing is uniquely focused on leveraging collective assets and resources to invest in initiatives intended to create inclusive, local economic growth to help address local issues of health and well-being. Collaborative partners invest a small percentage of their investment portfolios with the understanding that financial returns will be minimal or modest, although the impact on communities can be sizable. Pooling resources allows even partners with limited financial resources, such as many hospitals, to contribute to impact investing initiatives. Healthcare anchor collaboratives often combine place-based investment initiatives with community giving to maximize investment or engage in opportunities that would not otherwise be feasible.

Place-based investment strategies include low-interest loans, lines of credit, or equity capital to support affordable housing initiatives, development of multiuse facilities (buildings that house CBOs, health clinics, recreational facilities, childcare centers, arts and cultural activities, healthy food markets, etc.), and commercial development (e.g., improvements to storefronts), among other projects. Because both an insufficient supply of housing overall and a lack of affordable housing are among the nation's most critical problems,[6] a large number of anchor collective investments are dedicated to housing solutions. These include financing new construction, renovation of existing properties, and restoration of abandoned properties to create affordable housing, sometimes in conjunction with health and hospital systems' recruitment and retention initiatives, with priority given to the workforce of anchor organizations.

Anchor collaboratives often work with community development financial institutions, community development corporations, and neighborhood and regional associations on impact investing initiatives. Given the complexities and regulations associated with investing, as well as with the strategies for place-based investing in areas such as housing or real estate development, it is essential to obtain expert financial guidance when making investment plans and decisions.

## Volunteering and Advocacy

Many organizations across sectors encourage volunteering among their staff. Multisector collaboratives can work collectively to link volunteering needs and opportunities with their workforce, purchasing, and place-based investment strategies. In alignment with their health equity action plans, healthcare organizations should engage employees in identifying opportunities for volunteering in their own communities and may wish to consider incentives to support volunteering.

Anchor collaboratives can amplify their impact by working collectively to advocate for local, state, or national policies related to their initiatives and investments to support economic growth and improve community well-being. Advocacy efforts can engage broader coalitions and networks beyond the core partnerships, at the same time offering opportunities to extend the collaboratives' reach and impact.

## Funding Multisector Collaboratives

Anchor collaboratives fund their operations (staffing, meetings, events, data collection and management, contract management, etc.), initiatives, and programs (a job recruitment hub, a local supplier database, etc.) and support their place-based investments through a variety of mechanisms. Some anchor collaboratives require a one-time contribution from the core members to establish the collaborative and/or a commitment of ongoing support from the anchor institutions. Others fund basic functions through in-kind resources, while still others fund their work through allocations from state governments, city and county agencies, corporate philanthropy, community trusts, large philanthropic foundations, or matching fund campaigns.

The intention of multisector collaboratives committed to inclusive economic growth is to create lasting change. Decisions around funding should therefore reflect a commitment to, and plans to support, sustainability. Some anchor collectives have evolved to establish independent, community-led nonprofit (501[c][3]) entities, with the core anchor institutions providing ongoing guidance and participation in specific activities or initiatives of the new organization or, in some cases, serving as the organization's fiscal sponsor. However the collaborative is structured, the goal is for its work to be understood as part of a strategy for transformation.

Among the most promising and potentially powerful aspects of the anchor network movement are promoting collaboration over competition and championing collective impact over isolated organizational gains. Multisector partnership and collaborative strategies are essential for achieving health equity.

## Community Engagement

Community engagement can take many forms, from the Patient and Family Advisory Councils (PFACs) described in Chapter 3, to the participation of local communities in the design and delivery of antiracism and related trainings for healthcare organizations and hospital teams as described in Chapter 6, to partnering in the anchor collaborative initiatives we have summarized here. A large number of models and resources exist to guide community engagement strategies, all of which emphasize common core tenets; organizations must strive to build trust and develop robust relationships, recognizing that this will require time and concerted effort; respect the expertise and knowledge of communities, including their diverse perspectives and lived experience; refrain in any way from exploiting communities by extracting knowledge, data, or resources (including time) without their knowledge and consent; and commit to engaging in ways that are intended to benefit and support communities based on their priorities and preferences.[7,8]

Specific strategies for community engagement, like most of the initiatives described throughout this book, will be sensitive to local contexts as communities vary enormously. The core principles underlying meaningful engagement, nonetheless, remain constant. Before engaging in new efforts, organizations should identify existing community-engaged activities or community partnerships across departments and offices so as not to duplicate efforts or overburden community partners. It may be useful, where possible, to create a coordinated community engagement hub or dashboard to promote effective engagement throughout the organization.

## Payment and Reimbursement Models

Payors have an important role to play in advancing health equity. The fee-for-service model has produced a healthcare system that is expensive, fragmented, difficult to navigate, and ineffective in promoting health and optimizing health outcomes. The transition to value-based care is realigning financial incentives so that providers are held accountable for the quality of care delivered and for the outcomes achieved. When equity is embedded in the measurement of quality (as described in Chapter 2), this means that providers are held responsible for achieving equitable outcomes, rather than simply paid to deliver services.

This realignment of incentives has prompted many providers to actively address health-related social needs (HRSN), going far beyond the regulatory requirements to simply screen for HRSN and make referrals to address them. For example, bundling payments for operative procedures such as hip replacements has prompted some providers to send 30 days' worth of prepared meals to all patients after hospital discharge because proper nutrition is known to enhance recovery time and functional outcomes. A managed care organization may enter into a value-based contract with a healthcare provider, who in turn contracts with another organization to address HRSN. Under managed care or capitation arrangements, healthcare providers may arrange individualized care coordination with transportation services and patient navigators to assist high-risk patients in obtaining needed medical and social services.

Holding providers accountable for outcomes aligns the interests of providers and patients, and having providers share in lowered costs when unnecessary healthcare services and encounters are avoided has the effect of aligning the interests of providers and payors. As the clear benefits of addressing HRSN on improved outcomes and lower costs are repeatedly demonstrated, some fee-for-service payors have begun to directly reimburse social care providers for services rendered. Incorporating payment for their services is essential to the sustainability of social care providers and the establishment of a stable system for addressing HRSN, with the resultant benefits to all parties of improved outcomes and lower overall health costs.

## Payor-Financed Partnerships: Medicaid Delivery System Reform Incentive Payment (DSRIP)

Significant innovation in care delivery has been allowed within the Medicaid program through the use of Section 1115 Medicaid demonstration waivers, which offer states an avenue to test new approaches to "promote the objectives of the Medicaid program."[9] Several states, including New York, have used the Delivery System Reform Incentive Payment (DSRIP) mechanism to redesign the delivery of services to Medicaid beneficiaries. The Centers for Medicare & Medicaid Services (CMS) approved the initial New York State (NYS) DSRIP request in April 2014 to launch DSRIP-related programs through March 2020.

NYS DSRIP focused on reducing avoidable hospital use across the state by creating integrated delivery systems with value-based payment (VBP) arrangements. The entities responsible for creating and implementing the DSRIP projects were called "performing provider systems" (PPS): these partnerships included hospitals, federally qualified health clinics, primary care physicians, specialists, home care, skilled nursing homes, health homes, and behavioral health providers, as well as community-based organizations such as housing providers and social service agencies, so that the PPS had resources in the community to be able to address the social determinants of health.

Each PPS earned performance payments for achieving and reporting specific milestones and metrics. Through DSRIP, New York committed to shift 80% of all Medicaid managed care payments to value-based payment arrangements by March 2020, a goal that was reached over the course of the program, which included a planning year (year 0) and five years of DSRIP implementation.

After the conclusion of the program, evaluation by an independent evaluator[10] found that NYS DSRIP achieved substantial financial results, including an 18.1% reduction in potentially preventable readmission rates and a 26.1% reduction in potentially preventable admissions rates. Medicaid spending (per member per month) was virtually flat during a period of huge enrollment growth, rising only 1.9% over the five years of the program. There were significant reductions in hospital spending along with increased spending in ambulatory care, pharmacy, and long-term care. DSRIP also yielded significant statewide improvements in quality measures, including primary care quality and patient experience, timely access, care transitions, and system integration. The majority of the 25 performing provider systems improved on almost all performance measures, and surveys of PPS staff, healthcare and social care providers, and community leaders observed numerous successes, including stronger and more effective care collaboration, reduction of barriers between physical and behavioral health, cultural shifts to focus on population health and social determinants of health, opportunities for innovation, and investments in local infrastructure and workforce needs.

One of the most ambitious efforts ever attempted, NYS DSRIP made an $8 billion investment that involved millions of Medicaid members and more than 80,000 providers. Its successes benefited not only the payors but also the millions of members who use the healthcare system. DSRIP offers a blueprint for how to drive large-scale change by incentivizing local, place-based collaboratives of health and social care providers to improve population-level outcomes and accelerate the move to value-based care. In 2024, the state launched a new initiative to create sustainable social care networks to address health-related social needs through the New York Health Equity Reform (NYHER) 1115 Waiver program, which will also address workforce issues as well as behavioral health services.[11]

## Summary

1. Engage in multisector partnerships that promote collaboration over competition and collective impact over isolated organizational gains to alter the conditions created by decades of disinvestment and neglect in urban and rural communities across the country.
2. Advance the anchor role or mission in a collective effort to provide jobs and purchasing services, as well as to deliver health care. Hospitals and health systems have an important role to play in dismantling the policies, practices, and structures that created and have perpetuated health inequities.
3. Explore opportunities to implement the Healthcare Anchor Network's impact strategies—workforce, purchasing, investing—as a useful way to organize collaborative approaches to fuel economic growth and community wealth building.
4. Amplify the impact of collaborative networks by advocating for local, state, and national policies to support economic growth and improve community well-being.
5. Employ community engagement strategies that foster trust and the building of robust relationships, while respecting the expertise and knowledge of communities and their diverse perspectives.
6. Advocate for the development of value-based payor models that hold healthcare providers accountable for equitable outcomes and which can drive multisector collaborations that improve health and address HRSN.

## SPOTLIGHT

### Investing in Healthy Neighborhoods

*What creates the greatest impact for the community is having a seat at the table, deciding where resources will be directed, and activating their vision for what it means to build healthy neighborhoods.*

Ayesha Jako, MAM; Executive Director, West Side United

Residents of West Garfield Park and their neighbors in Chicago's downtown Loop area live five miles and a lifetime apart. A 14-year gap in life expectancy separates them. This disparity has been determined by so many others: stark inequities in median household income, educational attainment, and access to food, employment, financial services, and health care. A largely Black community (91.9% Black residents compared to 28.4% in Chicago overall), the West Garfield Park corridor has suffered from disinvestment and economic deterioration for decades—but that's about to change.[12]

The Sankofa Wellness Village (the Village), a multiuse, multiblock project, is set to bring an award-winning Federally Qualified Health Center (Erie Family Health Centers), a grocery store, a café, a credit union, the first arts facility in the neighborhood (MAAFA Center for Arts and Activism), and The K Entrepreneurial Hub (curated by Project Forward and Nation Builders) to the corridor, along with a gym and fitness facilities run by the YMCA and a rooftop terrace and community gardens. The Village is an initiative of the Garfield Park Rite to Wellness Collaborative. The office and services of West Side United (WSU), a member of the collaborative, will be located in the main building, including its workforce and community investment programs. Equal Hope, which provides breast and cervical cancer screening, patient navigation, outreach, and education, will also be housed there, helping to address one of WSU's "drivers of life expectancy" priorities (cardiometabolic disease, cancer, infant mortality, opioid overdose, and homicide). Rush University Medical Center will operate a comprehensive wellness center and coordinate a community health worker hub in the Village.

WSU was launched in 2018 as an anchor healthcare collaborative of six hospitals, including Rush, with the goal of reducing the life expectancy gap for residents of the West Side's 10 neighborhoods. When the COVID-19 pandemic demanded an urgent, coordinated response, the organization co-convened the city of Chicago's Racial Equity Rapid Response Team, which provided personal protective equipment (PPE), vaccination, testing and treatment, and education to the city's most affected neighborhoods. The organization, now an independent 501(c)(3), has since coalesced 100 technical, economic vitality, education, healthcare, and neighborhood partners, and through its multisector initiatives has supported highly impactful workforce, local purchasing, and career pathways projects. The founding hospitals have hired more than 4,000 West Side residents for open positions, and WSU partners have spent upward of $200 million with West Side vendors.

Re-industrialization projects of the size and scope of Sankofa Wellness Village require a sizeable investment, says WSU's executive director, Ayesha Jaco. But once partnerships are operationalized, there is so much that can be accomplished together. The Garfield Park Rite to Wellness Collaborative partnered with The Community Builders, Inc., Third Entity, and Moody Nolan, the largest Black-owned architectural design firm in the country, whose mission is to dismantle racism within its firm and in the world, to build the Sankofa Wellness Village. The project is funded by multiple sources, including new market tax credits and community development grants, and the prestigious Pritzker Traubert Chicago Prize, a $10 million award.

The Village will serve as a kind of studio for the Rush University Medical Center's BMO Institute for Health Equity, which is establishing an institutional data warehouse to support its research. "We have an opportunity to look at what is happening at the individual and community levels in terms of impacts on health and to ask *what are the difference makers?*" says the Institute's director, John Rich, MD. To measure its progress and success, WSU has developed a multitiered measurement framework that ties individual initiatives to population-wide metrics. Although the term Sankofa, which comes from West Africa, means "to go back for what is lost or forgotten," WSU is also looking ahead, considering the development of affordable housing projects in the area surrounding the Village and new economic partnerships among its hospital partners and others to create more jobs with family-sustaining wages.[13,14]

*As healthcare organizations, we have to shift power, earn trust, serve as honest brokers, and hold ourselves accountable for the long-term. This is what we mean by antiracist practice.* John Rich, MD, MPH, Inaugural Director, Rush BMO Institute for Health Equity, Rush University Medical Center

---

## Suggested Reading and Resources

American Planning Association. Planning and Community Health, Plan 4Health. Accessed January 21, 2025. https://www.planning.org/nationalcenters/health/

Center for Community Investment. Accessed January 19, 2025. https://centerforcommunityinvestment.org

The Democracy Collaborative. Community Wealth Building. Accessed January 19, 2025. https://www.democracycollaborative.org/community-wealth-building

Erickson D. Making missing markets: Strategic directions. Federal Reserve Bank of New York. November 2024. https://www.newyorkfed.org/medialibrary/media/outreach-and-education/household-financial-well-being/reports/2024/making-missing-markets

Healthcare Anchor Network. Activating place-based partnerships for equitable economic development: A playbook for collaboratives. Healthcare Anchor Network. May 2024. https://anchorcollaboratives.healthcareanchor.network/

MARGA, Inc. Anchor Institutions Task Force Anchor Partnerships Database. Accessed January 19, 2025. https://www.margainc.com/initiatives/anchor-institution-community-partnerships

National Academy of Medicine. Assessing Meaningful Community Engagement: A Conceptual Model to Advance Health Equity Through Transformed

Systems for Health. February 14, 2022. https://nam.edu/assessing-meaning ful-community-engagement-a-conceptual-model-to-advance-health-equity-t hrough-transformed-systems-for-health/

Rush University System for Health. Anchor mission playbook: New learnings and findings in anchor mission execution. Healthcare Anchor Network. October 9, 2024. https://healthcareanchor.network/2024/10/anchor-mission-playbook-new-learnings-findings-in-anchor-mission-execution/

We the World. Healthcare Transformation. Accessed December 25, 2024. https://weintheworld.org/resource_category/healthcare-transformation/

## References

1. Harker P, Diamond P, Reed D. Anchor impact: Understanding the role of higher education and hospitals in regional economies. Federal Reserve Bank. September 2022. https://www.philadelphiafed.org/-/media/FRBP/Assets/CommunityDevelopment/Reports/anchor-economy-report-92022.pdf
2. Federal Reserve Bank. Anchor Economy Dashboard. Accessed January 25, 2025. https://www.philadelphiafed.org/surveys-and-data/community-development-data/anchor-economy-dashboard
3. The Healthcare Anchor Network. Accessed January 25, 2025. https://healthcareanchor.network
4. MARGA, Inc. Anchor Institutions Task Force Anchor Partnerships Database. Accessed January 19, 2025. https://www.margainc.com/initiatives/anchor-institution-community-partnerships
5. National Academies of Sciences, Engineering, and Medicine. *Economic Systems as a Structural Driver of Population Health Through the Lens of Partnerships: Proceedings of a Workshop & #8212; in Brief.* National Academies Press; 2025. https://doi.org/10.17226/28879
6. National Low Income Housing Coalition. The Gap: A Shortage of Affordable Homes. March 2024. https://nlihc.org/gap
7. Robert Wood Johnson Foundation. Transformational Community Engagement to Advance Health Equity. January 2023. https://www.rwjf.org/en/insights/our-research/2023/01/transformational-community-engagement-to-advance-health-equity.htm
8. National Academy of Medicine. Assessing Meaningful Community Engagement: A Conceptual Model to Advance Health Equity Through Transformed Systems for Health. February 14, 2022. https://nam.edu/assessing-meaningful-community-engagement-a-conceptual-model-to-advance-health-equity-through-transformed-systems-for-health/
9. NY State Department of Health. Delivery System Reform Incentive Program (DSRIP). Accessed February 13, 2025. https://www.health.ny.gov/health_care/medicaid/redesign/dsrip/
10. Helgerson Solutions Group, LLC. Blueprint for Change: DSRIP's Independent Evaluator Finds Program Success, Goals Reached. Accessed March 11, 2025. https://www.hsg.global/insights/dsrips-independent-evaluator-finds-

program-a-success#:~:text=DSRIP%20successes%20observed%20by%20these,investments%20in%20local%20infrastructure%20and
11. NY State Department of Health. Medicaid Waiver Information Page. Accessed March 13, 2025. https://www.health.ny.gov/health_care/medicaid/redesign/medicaid_waiver_1115.htm
12. Community Data Snapshot. West Garfield Park. Chicago Metropolitan Agency for Planning. Accessed October 31, 2024. http://cmap.illinois.gov/wp-content/uploads/dlm_uploads/West-Garfield-Park.pdf
13. Ansell DA, Oliver-Hightower D, Goodman LJ, Lateerf DO, Johnson TJ. Health equity as a system strategy: The Rush University Medical Center framework. *NEJM Catalyst*. 2021; 2(5):1–19. doi: 10.1056/cat.20.0674
14. West Side United. Accessed October 31, 2024. https://westsideunited.org/

# Epilogue

Change is never easy. Throughout this book, we have endeavored to provide you with information, insights, and actionable advice to guide the transformation of health care by creating equitable, antiracist healthcare organizations. We hope that we have also inspired you to undertake the difficult work of scrutinizing every aspect of your organization to understand how racism is operating and the even more difficult challenge of dismantling the racism that you find embedded in organizational structures, processes, and policies.

We began with recommendations to support the design and implementation of a comprehensive antiracism action plan or road map to help navigate organizational change, from building a coalition or task force of leaders and staff from all levels throughout the organization who will identify priorities and develop the action plan to creation of an evaluation framework for assessing progress. Robust action plans will include, at a minimum, assessments of and recommendations for transforming patient care; development, training, and engagement of the workforce; application of an equity lens to business operations; the engagement of patients and communities in this important work; and development of the multisector partnerships and collaborations that will be key to advancing health equity. We have emphasized the need from the outset, and across every phase of the work, for accurate data, the inclusion of perspectives from individuals throughout the organization, transparency, and accountability.

The delivery of care is an immense, complex undertaking. We have focused in this book on several fundamental aspects of care delivery in the context of health equity. We encourage readers to view these essential strategies as a starting point that could be followed by comprehensive consideration of the specific policies and practices that impact access to and quality of care and are relevant to their organizations.

As a critical first step, we have described embedding equity into quality measurement with the accurate collection of patient data on race, ethnicity, and preferred language (REL), the development of REL capture-rate dashboards, and subsequent analysis of population health disparities. This work begins with the assessment of existing quality metrics, including both outcomes and process measures, which sets the stage for the types of questions and analyses that will allow for identification of disparities and inequities in care delivery.

An antiracist approach to transforming care demands that we identify and respond to health-related social needs (HRSN), not only in the context of inequitable access to health care, but also with regard to long-standing inequities in access to, as well as the distribution of, fundamental material and social resources. We consider the collection of HRSN data an important corollary to the collection of REL data and outlined both mandatory and more expansive screening options for social determinants of health and HRSN, as well as the subsequent linking of patients to health system–based or community-based resources to address these needs in more than a perfunctory way. We discussed the promise and perils of using community-level data on social determinants to understand and address patients' social risks and needs. The current regulations pertaining to screening for HRSN may be subject to change as national policies and guidelines in regulatory agencies are shaped by the current and future administrations. The recommendations we have outlined in this book will remain pertinent, and perhaps all the more so, if current requirements or guidelines for screening are altered or eliminated.

As we hope we have made clear, screening for HRSN is both of limited value and unjust if healthcare organizations do not also endeavor to address the needs identified. We have suggested a few of the many on-site and community-based resources that can be promoted or developed to connect patients and their families to support and services. Here, again, we urge readers to explore other models for partnering across their organizations and with local community-based organizations, faith-based organizations, and public agencies to respond to patients' HRSN. As we have emphasized throughout this book, we must collectively address the larger structural issues that have created vast and disproportionate social deficits. But in so doing, we cannot lose sight of our patients' immediate needs.

We also considered communication, specifically attention to language preference and health literacy, as critical to embedding equity into care. These components of care delivery continue to be underappreciated, underdeveloped, and underresourced. Our recommendations around the provision of high-quality language assistance or interpreting and translation services, and for the creation of materials and methods that will accommodate the low levels of health literacy that are prevalent across the country, are not meant to be aspirational. These services and programs are underfunded nearly everywhere and are often underutilized even where they do exist and are reimbursed. Enforceable national policies and hyperlocal solutions are needed in this area, and we hope our brief consideration of these issues will inspire readers to explore options and opportunities to promote and develop equitable communication strategies as integral to the delivery of equitable care.

Our discussion of bias and discrimination in care delivery focused on the need to eliminate race-biased algorithms used for clinical decision-making, such as estimated glomerular filtration rate (eGFR), which is used to assess kidney function, and the fact that flawed inclusion of race in the calculation resulted in inaccuracies, with devastating consequences for many Black patients. As we explained, a number of algorithms that include race as a factor in decisions about care are currently under review and research is ongoing. We expect this critical work to continue given the increasing use of algorithms for clinical decision-making and the impact on patient outcomes. This is particularly true of artificial intelligence algorithms and tools, where detecting and eliminating bias is of immense importance, as their incorporation into all aspects of health care accelerates. However, we emphasize that the appropriate consideration of race and ethnicity and other personal characteristics in medical decision-making about diagnostic and treatment options is essential to providing effective and equitable care.

In considering the elimination of bias and discrimination in care delivery, we also looked briefly at issues of practice segregation. Segregation in ambulatory healthcare settings takes several forms, including physically separate sites with different staffing and resources for different groups of patients, as well as internally segregated teaching practices where attending physicians may see commercially insured patients while students, residents, and fellows see Medicaid and uninsured patients. This is another complex issue that will most certainly be impacted by evolving changes in payor models and will continue to require attention and thoughtful analysis across different settings.

These days, it is hard to imagine discussion of equitable care delivery without considering emerging digital trends, an area with enormous implications for equity. We looked at digital health strategies, including online patient portals to their electronic health records (EHR), telehealth initiatives, and remote patient monitoring; these are rapidly evolving areas with great potential either for exclusion and discrimination or for inclusion and equity, depending on their design and distribution. Here, again, national and local policies and regulations will influence and guide access and affordability, and it will be important for healthcare organizations to advocate for inclusion of their patients and local communities in digital health advances and innovation.

An organization's workforce is a core component of any racial health equity action plan. We have described antiracist practices for human resources, including the recruitment, hiring, and retention of a workforce that mirrors the region and communities it serves, and the development of inclusive workplace cultures. We considered strategies for engagement in local schools and community organizations to support both interest in the health sciences professions more generally and recruitment for the organization, equitable design of performance metrics and pay equity practices, mentorship and leadership development programs to enhance retention, and equitable strategies for enhancing employee engagement. Our recommendations for creating and sustaining an antiracist, inclusive workplace culture include various training themes and programs for leaders and employees at all levels with the aim to reduce bias and encourage allyship. We realize that these programs may be challenging to initiate or sustain at a time when race consciousness may be misunderstood, under attack, or both, but we hope that organizations will want to support leaders and employees in developing an actively antiracist environment.

Finally, we have reiterated across multiple chapters the importance of developing multisector partnerships and engaging with local communities as integral to comprehensive health equity action plans, from the development of co-located services, to diversification of the supply chain, to place-based investing. We described organizational strategies to stand up formal programs and systems to engage local suppliers and vendors and to ensure successful, mutually beneficial partnerships. We recommended strategies for identifying new vendors, working collaboratively with other organizations to maximize opportunities and resources, and tracking progress. Here, again, an evolving national landscape may create uncertainty about the most effective methods for implementing supplier diversity programs, but excellent models and resources exist to help guide the way. Cultivating productive relationships with local businesses is a winning strategy on many levels.

Our book concludes with a look at the role of healthcare organizations as anchor institutions—employers with a significant financial stake in their local communities and an obligation to contribute to the region's economic health and well-being—and with a brief consideration of payor models. Health and hospital systems have partnered with organizations from multiple sectors—government, industry, the nonprofit sector, finance, philanthropy, and education—to invest in housing, workforce development, multiuse facilities, and locally owned businesses that serve to improve or revitalize their communities and advance health equity goals.

Last, payors play an undeniably important role in advancing health equity to drive accountability for health outcomes. We looked at one innovative model, the Delivery System Reform Incentive Payment (DSRIP), which created multisector partnerships to deliver value-based care and was shown to be effective in improving a number of health outcomes while reducing the associated costs of care in a large state. Payor models and reimbursement schemes will most assuredly continue to be an area where attention, innovation, and advocacy to ensure equity will be required, especially in the context of what may be dramatic shifts in national and state budgets for covered care.

Being antiracist means actively opposing policies, behaviors, and beliefs that perpetuate racist ideas and actions, whenever and wherever you see them. Doing this work takes courage, effort, and persistence. There will be times when you feel overwhelmed, especially when others try to persuade you that the changes you seek are unnecessary or go too far. But there will also be times when it is clear to you that the changes you are making will benefit both your institution and the patients you serve. Those times will make you proud and will give you the energy to continue to work toward equity. It is not enough to know better—we must do better. It is not likely or even realistic that you will be able to do everything at once, but do not let that keep you from doing anything at all. Start where you are, do what you can, and find colleagues and allies to help you make sustained change.

The Spotlight stories we have included throughout this book represent just a few of the many healthcare organizations across every region of the country that have begun this difficult work; many have been committed to achieving health equity for a long time. Their strategies reflect rigor, innovation, and willingness to question—and sometimes, when necessary, to disrupt the status quo. The leaders of these healthcare organizations and hospital systems understand that achieving organizational excellence, economic vitality, and health equity are inseparable goals. These organizations center the voices of patients and embrace their critical role in the life of the neighborhoods and communities they serve. They know that change may be slow but believe, nonetheless, that it is possible to recognize the urgency of the situation while taking the necessary steps and devoting the essential resources—time, funds, and attention—to ensure enduring solutions. We are confident that even as the national landscape shifts, as policies remain unclear or in flux, and as issues that once seemed settled may now become muddled or unclear, committed leaders and a healthcare workforce dedicated to the best health and well-being of our patients, and to society as a whole, will persist and will prevail.

# Index

*For the benefit of digital users, indexed terms that span two pages (e.g., 52–53) may, on occasion, appear on only one of those pages.*